DREAM HIKES
COAST TO COAST

Dear Karla,

Happy Birthday! Hope you
have a fabulous day. You
deserve it.   Thank you for being
a great friend, neighbor and
inspiration to be a better person.

♡ Tyler, Leslie, Kyle

2017

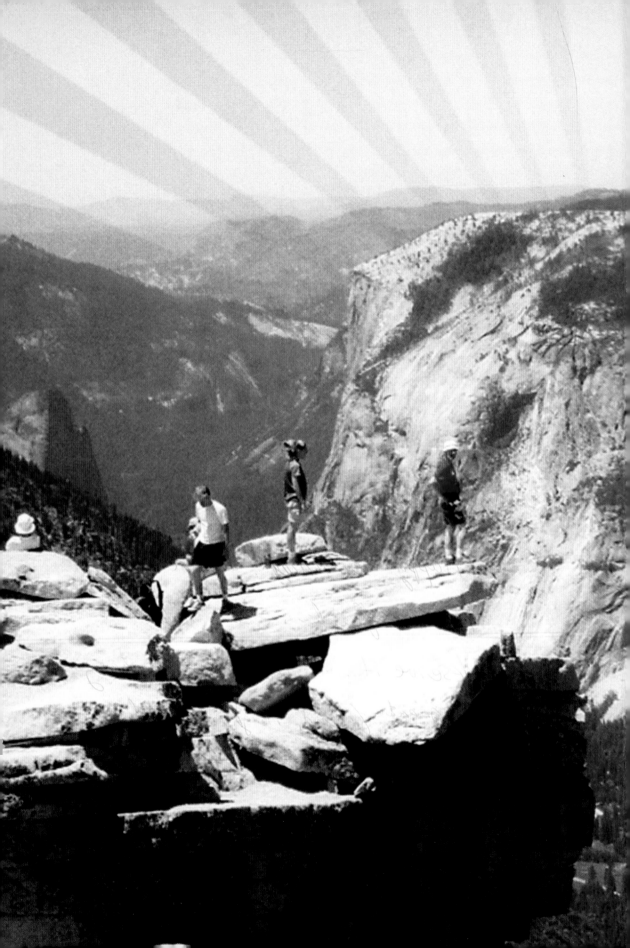

DREAM HIKES
COAST TO COAST

BY JACK BENNETT

Your Guide to America's Most Memorable Trails

MENASHA RIDGE PRESS
www.menasharidge.com

Dream Hikes Coast to Coast:
Your Guide to America's Most Memorable Trails

Published by Menasha Ridge Press

Distributed by Publishers Group West

Manufactured in China

First edition, first printing

ISBN 978-0-89732-710-7

Cover design by Scott McGrew

Text design by Travis Bryant

Front cover photo by Jack Bennett *(The author standing atop the "Visor" of Half Dome in Yosemite National Park)*

Mt. Katahdin photo on page 191 by Ron Chase

Author photo by Sandy Dulla

All other photos by Jack Bennett and Mary Fran Bennett

Maps by Scott McGrew and Jack Bennett

Indexing by Rich Carlson

Menasha Ridge Press

PO Box 43673

Birmingham, AL 35243

www.menasharidge.com

DISCLAIMER

This book is meant only as a guide to select trails in the United States and does not guarantee hiker safety in any way—you hike at your own risk. Neither Menasha Ridge Press nor Jack Bennett is liable for property loss or damage, personal injury, or death that result in any way from accessing or hiking the trails described in this book. Be aware that hikers have been injured in these areas. Be especially cautious when walking on or near boulders, steep inclines, and drop-offs, and do not attempt to explore terrain that may be beyond your abilities. To help ensure an enjoyable hike, please carefully read the introduction to this book and familiarize yourself thoroughly with the areas you intend to visit before venturing out by asking questions, preparing for the unforeseen, and obtaining further safety information and guidance from additional sources. Familiarize yourself with current weather reports, maps of the area you intend to visit, and any relevant park regulations.

CONTENTS

Dedication

This book is dedicated to my remarkable family and their endurance of my whims. They always gave me support, and often accompanied me even when they knew that the misadventure I had planned was a bad idea.

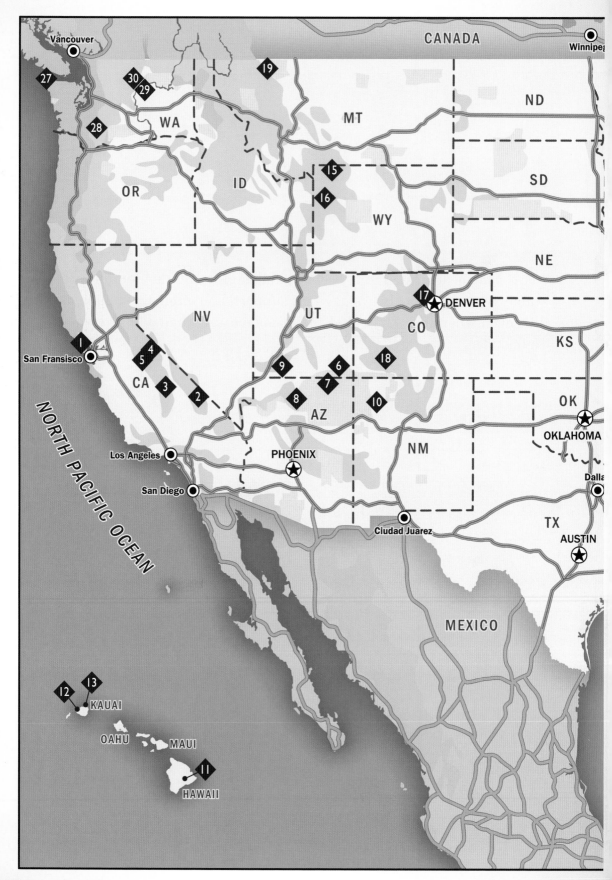

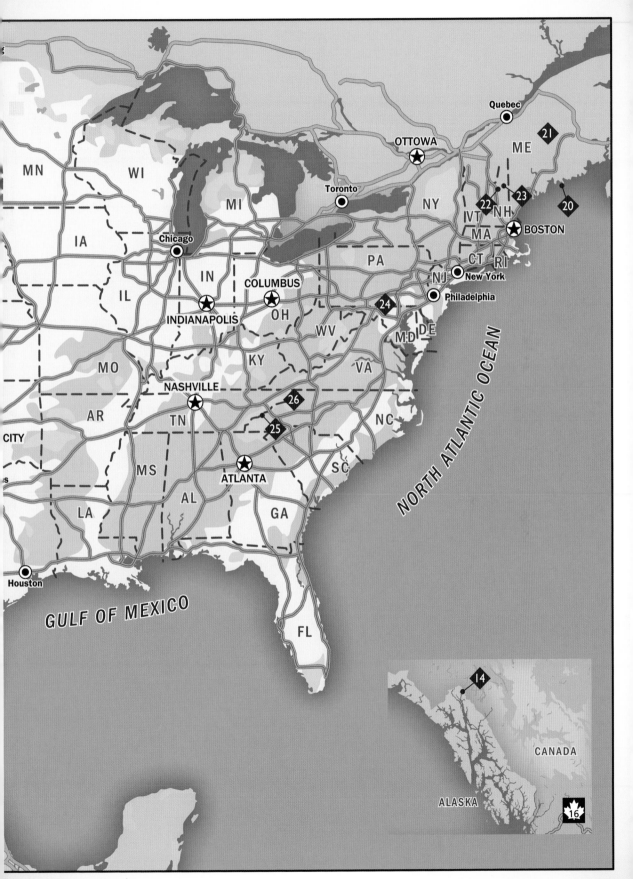

Acknowledgments

I would like to first acknowledge the Highpointers Club, especially those members who returned my surveys. Not only did they recommend the hikes for this book, but many also wrote detailed descriptions of favorite hikes, copied pages out of guidebooks, and sent maps to help me with this project. Thank you to the many park rangers and information attendants who gave me good on-site advice before beginning a hike.

I also owe a special debt of gratitude to Dan Bennett and especially my wife, Mary Fran Bennett, for the many hours they spent proofreading my writing. It was definitely a labor of love, and I love them for it.

About the Author

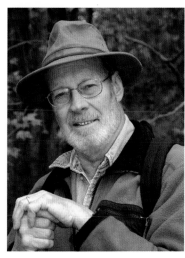

Jack Bennett is a lifelong runner, hiker, and mountain climber. He has completed six full marathons and one mountain marathon. He is currently a member of the Highpointers Club and the American Alpine Club. In 1990 Jack became the 12th person to climb to the highest points of all 50 U.S. states. In 1998 he became the first person to climb the Highpoints of Canada—the highest point of all 13 Canadian Provinces and Territories. Jack is an official Guinness World Record holder for this achievement, which has never been repeated.

In 1999 Jack published the book *Not Won In a Day, Climbing Canada's Highpoints,* available from Rocky Mountain Books. The book is a combination guidebook and adventure story about his experiences climbing the wild and challenging Highpoints of Canada.

In his professional life, Jack owns his own research and development company, J.E. Bennett Consultants, Inc., and has authored 34 issued U.S. patents, about 70 technical publications and book chapters, as well as a few entries in *American Alpine Journal.* He has been fortunate enough in his work to be able to finance his *real* passion: hiking and climbing the beautiful and fantastic wild places of America with his family.

Preface

I have traveled extensively in America throughout my life and have a lifelong love affair with its natural wonders. I love America's majestic mountains, secret canyons, rockbound coasts, thundering waterfalls, waving grasslands, and peaceful forests. My wife Mary Fran and I also love road trips where we only stay one to three days in each place, taking in as much as we can in a limited period of time.

We love to hike America's many wonderful trails. Often the most memorable sights cannot be seen from the highway—the longest stone arch, the highest natural bridge, the best-preserved Anasazi ruins, the mysterious Zion Narrows, and any number of unforgettable views. When planning a new road trip, I have always tried to include a few hikes. But here I encountered a problem: Which hikes should I include? I consulted various hiking guidebooks but still couldn't figure out which hikes were best for our limited schedule. Guidebooks seldom compared hikes objectively, and none compared hikes on a national scope.

So in April 2000 I set off on a quest to identify and actually hike our country's best hikes—the Dream Hikes of America. It was a quest that would last seven years and take Mary Fran and me on an unforgettable journey. By the end of this journey, I had memories to last a lifetime: I had been stuck in quicksand, nearly trapped by a flash flood, stalked by a grizzly bear, and faced all manner of severe weather. But I had also experienced the splendor and wonder of America's great natural treasures. I want to convey to the readers of this guidebook not simply directions, distances, and contacts but also what each hike looked, smelled, and felt like; the animals I saw; and the weather I experienced. Each one of the hikes in this book, like the patches of a beautiful quilt, will forever be a part of my life.

Introduction

HOW THE HIKES WERE SELECTED

To select America's *Dream Hikes Coast to Coast,* I first turned to the Highpointers Club, a 2,700-member mix of mountain climbers, hikers, and list keepers. The principal goal for each Highpointer is to ascend the highest point in every state. To accomplish this goal they travel extensively, and most are also familiar with hikes across the breadth of America. Before traveling to a particular region of the country, I sent 20 to 25 surveys to Highpointers in that region. In the survey I asked the club member to identify the top five hikes in his or her region. Nearly all of my surveys were completed and returned to me.

For hikes to be nominated, I needed to establish criteria. For example, I asked for hikes that could be completed in a single day. For me, that restricts hikes to between 5 and 20 miles. Nominating the Appalachian Trail, for example, was not allowed. The hikes were also to be on maintained, or at least well-traveled, trails. Off-trail rambling was not considered. Solitude was not a criterion. The best hikes are, unfortunately, not well-kept secrets, and the finest trails in America are often congested. Those seeking solitude would be well advised to look elsewhere. Also, geographic fit was not a consideration—the trails selected are the best America has to offer regardless of location. States like California, Washington, and Hawaii have five, four, and three hikes, respectively (sorry, Kansas). Finally, and above all else, the hikes should have some quality that makes them special . . . in a word, memorable.

The results of my surveys were intriguing. Sometimes there was a remarkable consensus, such as the resounding choice of Franconia

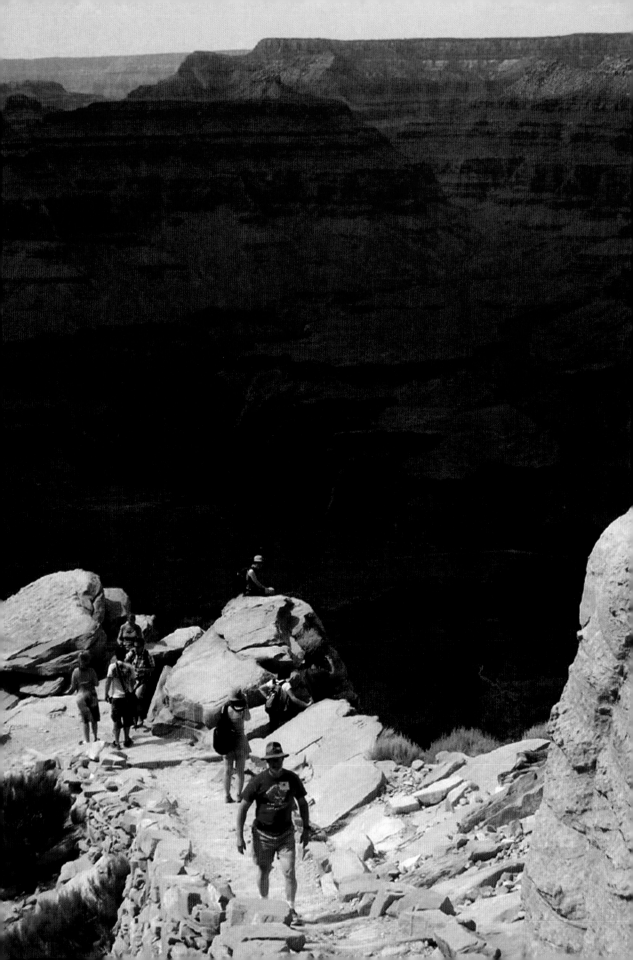

Ridge as the top hike in New England. Sometimes there was little agreement, such as for the best hikes in the Pacific Northwest. Although there were trends, everyone in the Northwest seemed to have a different favorite, and a large number of hikes were nominated. I credit this result with the large number of excellent hikes in that region. Regardless, by the end of the survey process I had several hikes in each region with 2 to 12 nominations. I then traveled to each region and walked the top hikes myself for final consideration.

The hikes with the most votes never disappointed me, but sometimes hikes with more than one vote did not meet expectations. For example, Lassen Peak in California had little appeal for me other than a good view at the top. My own opinion in comparing the hike to other candidates was the final arbitrator.

Because of the nature of the survey population, hikes nominated were biased toward mountain hikes. I wanted to identify the best hikes in America, not just the top mountain hikes. To prevent this domination, I had to more heavily weight other types of hikes: canyon hikes, waterfall hikes, forest hikes, coastal hikes, historical hikes, and others. I also made an effort to include the most significant natural features: the deepest canyon, the highest waterfall, the biggest tree, the best-preserved ruin, and the most beautiful and best-recognized features in the country. It is perhaps not surprising that 23 of the 30 hikes in this book are located in national parks, national monuments, or national historic parks.

At the end of this process, I had a list that identified my top 30 Dream Hikes in America. Another person's list would be different, just as every person's experience and viewpoint are different. This fact was made clear by the results of my surveys. But I do believe that anyone who hikes this selection will encounter the very best America has to offer.

THE BEST OF THE BEST

Since I personally experienced all of the hikes in this book, I am in a unique position to evaluate the best hikes in each category. This information is found nowhere else, and I hope it will be valuable to readers. See my list for the best of the best on the next page:

Best Hike in the Northeast	Franconia Ridge
Best Hike in the Southeast	Roan Mountain (in June)
Best Hike in the Northwest	Cascade Pass–Sahale Arm Trail
Best Canyon Hikes	(tie) Zion Narrows and South Kaibab–Bright Angel Loop
Best Coastal Hike	Kalalau Trail
Best Historical Hike	Billy Yank Trail
Best Waterfall Hike	Yosemite Falls Trail
Best Mountain Hikes	(tie) Cascade Pass and Amphitheater Lake Trails
Best Wildflower Hikes	(tie) Highline Trail–Loop Trail and Roan Mountain (in June)
Special Mention	Half Dome

HOW TO USE THIS GUIDEBOOK

The Overview Map and Map Key

The overview map (pages viii–ix) can be used to assess the location of each hike. Each hike's number appears on the overview map and in the Table of Contents. The hike number also appears at the top of each hike profile for easy reference.

Regional Maps

The book is organized by region as indicated in the Table of Contents. Prefacing each regional section is an overview map of that region. The regional map provides more detail than the overview map, giving you a more exact location of the hike.

Trail Maps

Each hike contains a detailed map that shows the trailhead, route, significant features, and topographic landmarks such as creeks and peaks.

Elevation Profiles

Corresponding directly to the trail map, each hike contains a detailed elevation profile. The elevation profile provides a quick look at the trail from the side, enabling you to visualize how the trail rises and falls. The elevation profile shows both the total elevation gain, as well as the steepness of the trail, and provides an easy assessment of the hike's climbing difficulty.

Trailhead Coordinates

The location of each trailhead is provided in two formats: latitude-longitude and UTM. Latitude-longitude coordinates locate a point north or south (latitude) of the 0° line known as the equator and west (longitude) of the 0° meridian line that passes through Greenwich, England. Latitude and longitude coordinates are each shown in degrees north of the equator or west of the meridian line, minutes (each degree is divided into 60 minutes), and seconds (each minute is divided into 60 seconds).

UTM coordinates locate a specific point on the earth using a grid method. The UTM convention used in this book is WGS84 (versus NAD27 or WGS83). The first field of the UTM coordinates contains a zone number and a zone letter. The zone number refers to one of 60 vertical zones, each zone being 6 degrees wide. The zone letter refers to one of 20 horizontal zones that span from 80 degrees south to 84 degrees north. The second field of the UTM coordinates, referred to as the easting number, indicates in meters how far east or west a point is from the central meridian of the zone. Increasing easting coordinates on the map indicate you are moving east. The final field in the UTM, referred to as the northing number, indicates in meters how far you are from the equator. Increasing northing coordinates indicate you are moving north.

For readers who own a GPS unit, the latitude-longitude or UTM coordinates provided for each hike trailhead may be entered into the GPS unit. A GPS unit is not required, however. All of the hikes contained in this book are relatively popular and well traveled, and the trailheads can be located from the Directions to the Trailhead and Trail Route provided in each hike profile and from local information.

Key At-a-Glance Information

DISTANCE The length of the hike from start to finish is provided. In some cases there may be options to shorten or extend the hike, but the mileage provided corresponds to the principal hike as described. If the route is an out-and-back, the distance provided refers to the total distance traveled to the end of the trail and then back to the trailhead.

The time needed to cover the total distance varies depending on terrain, elevation, trail and weather conditions, and a hiker's individual speed. The hike description always provides the time that I took to complete the hike, but that can be misleading. Sometimes I hiked slowly, taking in all the marvels of the trail. Sometimes I hiked fast, and sometimes too fast. A rule often used is to allow one hour for every 2 miles of trail, and add one hour for every 1,000 feet of elevation gained. This formula will usually be fairly accurate, except for unusual cases such as the Zion Narrows, where hiking in water slows the pace.

ELEVATION EXTREMES The highest and lowest elevations on the hike are presented as elevation extremes. This can be useful information, especially for hikes at high elevations such as Telescope Peak, Amphitheater Lake, Longs Peak, and Chicago Basin. High elevation takes a toll on the body, and those who attempt these hikes should properly acclimatize themselves. This is best done by training at higher altitudes and by sleeping as high as possible prior to the hike. There have been times when I suffered considerably by ignoring the need to acclimatize.

TOTAL ELEVATION GAIN The total elevation gain is the sum of all the rises in elevation for the entire hike, both out and back. Elevation gain adds greatly to the total effort needed for a hike and is a very important factor for planning. I have already mentioned that 1,000 feet of elevation gain will add about one hour to the hiking time, but the additional toll on the body can be more significant. For example, the Kalalau Trail on the coast of Kauai never rises to 800 feet above sea level, but the trail is almost never level. Total elevation gain of the Kalalau Trail is difficult to judge since there are countless small rises. The 2,750-foot total elevation gain provided is likely an underestimate, as the Kalalau Trail is extremely demanding.

DIFFICULTY The difficulty of each trail is listed as either easy, moderate, strenuous, or very strenuous. These are subjective terms and somewhat difficult to relate to. As you complete some of the hikes in this book, you will acquire a better impression of the meaning of these terms. Only hikers who are strong and fit and have trained adequately for the challenge should attempt the very strenuous hikes in this book.

USGS MAPS USGS Maps are topographic maps produced by the United States Geological Survey (USGS). A topographic map is a type of map characterized by large-scale detail and a quantitative representation of relief. Some hikers prefer to obtain USGS Maps for planning purposes, or for added safety when hiking. Topographic maps show topography, or land contours, by means of contour lines. Contour lines are curved lines that connect all points of the same altitude. Topographic maps can reveal important information. For example: sharp, pointed Vs are usually in stream valleys with the V pointing upstream (rule of Vs); closed loops represent hilltops, with the innermost loop the highest area (rule of Os); and close contour lines indicate a steep slope, while distant contour lines indicate a shallow slope.

The USGS produces several series of topographic maps that vary in scale and extent. The largest and best-known series is the 7.5-minute, 1:24,000 scale map bounded by two lines of latitude and two lines of longitude spaced 7.5 minutes apart. The 15-minute map, an older series, is bounded by two lines of latitude and two lines of longitude spaced 15 minutes apart. These maps are available on the Internet at a number of sites for affordable commercial and recreational use.

Hike Description

The description of the hike itself will be the most informative, and I hope the most interesting, part of this book. The hike description relates not only what I saw, experienced, and felt during my hike, but also what the next hiker is likely to encounter on that trail. Problems I experienced and lessons I learned, like my encounter with quicksand and flash flood on the trail to Keet Seel, will hopefully help to make the next hiker's walk safer and more enjoyable. I hope readers will find each hike, as it was for me, to be a deeply rewarding personal experience.

Directions to Trailhead and Trail Route

Directions to the trailhead, together with the trail map, should be sufficient to locate the trailhead without the use of GPS. With few exceptions, you can access the trailhead for every hike in this book with a two-wheel-drive passenger vehicle. Two trails, South Kaibab–Bright Angel Loop and Zion Narrows, must be accessed by bus shuttle. Chelan Lakeshore Trail can be accessed only by boat, and the trailhead for Chicago Basin is accessible only from the Durango-Silverton Narrow Gauge Railway. The last 1.4 miles of road to the Telescope Peak trailhead is suitable only for high-clearance, preferably four-wheel-drive vehicles. But in every case, locating and accessing the trailhead will not be difficult.

Directions for the trail route, together with the trail map, should be adequate for following the trail to its conclusion. The directions for the route should be carefully consulted at each trail junction. Almost all hikes in this book follow well-marked and maintained trails. Where the trail is not officially maintained, a well-worn path can still be discerned. Hikes that include sections of primitive trail include Tomales Point Trail, Amphitheater Lake–Teton Glacier Trail, Devils Garden Loop, Keet Seel, Zion Narrows, and Cascade Pass–Sahale Arm Trail.

Weather and Wildlife

I describe the weather for each hike's location at all times of the year for those who prefer to hike in seasons other than summer.

The animals I describe for each hike location are principally large mammals such as deer, elk, moose, bear, and so on. Small mammals, insects, amphibians, reptiles, and birds are not usually listed except for special cases, such as the California condors soaring over the Grand Canyon, feral chickens on the Waimea Canyon Loop, and rattlesnakes on the Chelan Lakeshore Trail.

Lodging and Camping

I have included information on campgrounds closest to the trailhead for each hike, as well as information on lodging, especially lodging I have found particularly enjoyable. I especially enjoy the historic national park lodges and stay in them whenever I can. The Old Faithful Inn (page 141), Granite Park Chalet (pages 172–173), LeConte Lodge (page 227–278), Bright Angel Lodge (page 84), and Zion Lodge (page 92) have provided me with many unforgettable nights. I enthusiastically recommend them all. More traditional hotels and motels in nearby towns are not described in detail.

Fees and Contacts

Finally, entrance and parking fees are presented as priced in 2009. Entrance fees, like everything else, can be expected to increase with time. Useful addresses and phone numbers are included, and Internet addresses (where more detailed information such as bear status or current trail conditions can be accessed) are also provided.

HIKING SAFETY

In the spring of 2003, a young couple came to seek my advice about climbing Mount d'Iberville, a remote and difficult mountain in northern Quebec. I spent a few hours describing access to the mountain, the various climbing routes, as well as the hazards involved. They left full of enthusiasm for the adventure ahead. In August of that year the young couple went north to climb Mount d'Iberville and died. The next year I led an expedition to help recover their bodies. The role I played in this tragedy haunts me to this day. Should I have asked more about their experience? Should I have better stressed the dangers of this wild and unforgiving place? Could I have done or said anything to prevent this tragedy? I never again want to ask myself these questions.

A few of the hikes in this book can be dangerous, especially if attempted in a single day. These include South Kaibab–Bright Angel Loop, Zion Narrows, Knife Edge of Mount Katahdin, Longs Peak Trail, and to a lesser extent Amphitheater Lake–Teton Glacier Trail, Half Dome, Telescope Peak Trail, and Kalalau Trail. Each of these hikes has unique hazards. Please carefully read the following sections on safety, make sure you completely understand the hazards of each hike, and fully prepare yourself for the mental and physical challenges ahead. YOUR SAFETY IS YOUR RESPONSIBILITY.

Weather

Many people in this country die from weather-related conditions each year. Several can be related to severe mountain weather. Storms can strike high mountains with little warning and unbelievable fury. Temperature and windchill can drop suddenly, rain can quickly soak clothing, and wind can knock you to the ground. Hikers are often reluctant to turn back short of their goal, even under such conditions. Always remember that safety lies below. Do not underestimate the danger of such storms, and turn back without shame before it's too late. Severe storms on mountains of the Southwest and Rocky Mountain West are common during the monsoon season, which generally lasts from late June until early September. Mornings frequently dawn clear during the monsoons, but clouds build during the day, and storms strike in the afternoon. For the hikes on Longs Peak, Amphitheater Lake–Teton Glacier, and Telescope Peak, start early, plan to summit before noon, and descend before afternoon thunderstorms build. Also, beware of mountain storms on the hikes to Chicago Basin, Half Dome, and Cascade Pass. Eastern mountains are not exempt from these dangers. The many hikers who have died on the slopes of Mount Washington, Mount Katahdin, and others in the Northeast are adequate testament to the fury of summer storms in New England.

Lightning is a common feature of high mountain storms. The summits of some sharp mountains are covered with glassy nodules from frequent lightning strikes. I was hiking with my family high on the summit ridge of Humphrey's Peak in Arizona when dark afternoon clouds quickly gathered, and our hair began to stand on end. Rather than descend, we huddled in a small rock cave while lightning crashed around us—a poor decision. We were lucky.

Deep in the canyons of the Southwest, flash floods from storms present another danger. Heavy rain falling on the slickrock of the mesas quickly funnels into slot canyons where water levels can rise several feet in a matter of minutes, sometimes with deadly consequences. Flash floods can be especially dangerous in the Zion Narrows, where a single flood once caught 26 climbers, drowning 5. Be aware of the weather forecast and do not hike the Zion Narrows if thunderstorms threaten.

Heat is another weather-related danger, particularly in the desert Southwest where many people die from dehydration and heat exhaustion each year. Heat is a particular hazard in the Grand Canyon, where temperatures in the inner gorge can be torrid, with daily highs averaging 106°F in July. Visitors hiking down into the canyon often fail to appreciate the effort needed to climb back up to the rim in stifling heat. As a result, about 250 people need to be evacuated by helicopter from the depths of the canyon each year. Do not attempt the South Kaibab–Bright Angel Loop hike, especially in summer, unless you fully appreciate the risk and are completely prepared for the challenge. Heat can also be a factor on the hikes to Keet Seel, Kalalau Trail, and Yosemite Falls Trail. Heat can even be a problem on shorter hikes such as Devils Garden Loop and Pueblo Alto Loop.

Clothing

Proper clothing is important for both comfort and safety. Wear clothing in layers, which can be either added or removed depending on weather conditions. On hikes where cold, wet weather threatens, remember "cotton kills." In such cases, choose a wool sweater and clothing made of synthetic fiber, such as polypropylene. Choose a warm stocking hat in cold weather and a broad sun hat for protection on hot, sunny days.

Carry raingear whenever rain is a possibility. Remember that getting soaked opens the door to hypothermia, which occurs when the amount of heat lost to the environment exceeds that produced by the body. When the core temperature of the body is sufficiently reduced, muscular and cerebral functions become impaired. Stages of hypothermia include shivering, loss of coordination, slow stumbling pace, mental sluggishness with slow thought and speech, severe muscle rigidity, and finally, unconsciousness and death. The best safeguard against hypothermia is preparation and your own intellect.

Proper footwear is also important. Sturdy hiking boots with solid ankle support have long been the footwear of choice, but lifting heavy hiking boots every step of the way for several miles can take an additional toll on energy. Most of the trails in this book have relatively smooth, well-maintained surfaces, and in such cases I recommend light running shoes. But you should still wear sturdy hiking boots when hiking trails where the terrain is rough, such as the Knife Edge of Mount Katahdin, Presidential Range Loop, Amphitheater Lake–Teton Glacier Trail, Longs Peak Trail, Cascade Pass–Sahale Arm Trail, and Chilkoot Trail. Wearing shoes without good support on these trails is to risk ankle injury and a painful limp back to the car.

Water

Be sure to carry sufficient water for the hike. Before hiking in hot weather, I hydrate thoroughly at the trailhead and then carry about a quart of fluid for every two hours of hiking (about 8 ounces of fluid per mile). My family and I once ran out of water on Devils Garden Loop, giving us a stern impression of the consequences of poor planning. The pleasures of hiking make carrying water a small price to pay to remain healthy.

I never drink water found along the trail unless absolutely necessary. The most common risk is Giardia, a nasty parasite that will leave you living in the bathroom with diarrhea, vomiting, and chills. Other parasites, such as E.coli and Cryptosporidium, are harder to kill than Giardia. Drinking water found on the Kalalau Trail can result in leptospirosis, a potentially fatal disease often mistaken for hepatitis. On overnight hikes, backpackers usually hit the trail prepared to purify water with either water purifiers or a number of commercially available tablets. I choose to take a small dropper bottle filled with common chlorine bleach solution, such as Clorox®. Treat every quart of clear water with five drops of bleach (for 15 ppm dose) and let it stand 20 minutes before using. Although slightly distasteful, chlorine is a reliable disinfectant, effective against a broad range of parasites and viruses.

Not Getting Lost

Getting lost should not be a problem for the hikes in this book. Your best safeguard against getting lost is your intellect. Whenever confronted with a trail junction, consult the trail route directions, think carefully, and if necessary, refer to your compass or GPS unit. When on a primitive trail, be on the alert constantly for painted trail marks or cairns that mark the way. Be especially cautious on the off-trail section of Amphitheater Lake–Teton Glacier Trail; when on the outward part of the hike, turn around occasionally and see what the return journey looks like. Pick out features and landmarks to help you find your way back.

For the longer hikes in this book, always tell someone of your plans and schedule. If you do become lost, remain calm and think your way back. Carefully retrace your steps until you again find yourself in familiar surroundings. If you do become hopelessly lost and have no idea how to continue, remain in place and wait for help. Consider carrying a whistle. It's more effective for signaling rescuers than your own voice.

Animal Hazards

The most common animal hazards you are likely to encounter on the trails in this book are bears and snakes. Snakes are possible but unlikely for several of the hikes in the Southwest and Rocky Mountain West. If you do see or hear a rattlesnake, leave it alone and give it a wide berth.

Bear sightings are far more likely. I have seen a total of seven bears on these hikes, and chances are good you will see some, too. I saw a mother black bear and two cubs on Alum Cave Bluff Trail. I also had a frightening encounter with a male grizzly bear on Highline Trail. The strategy is different for encounters with black and grizzly bears. For black bears, stand your ground and raise your arms to look large and intimidating. Do not run. Grizzly bears are very territorial, so looking aggressive is a bad idea. For grizzlies, most experts advise looking as submissive as possible. Turn sideways to present a low profile, lower your head, and do not make eye contact. Back away slowly if possible. The sound of the human voice is the best deterrent to bear encounters. Talk or sing when you are on the trail in bear country, especially when rounding a blind corner or making your way through brush. So-called "bear bells" are not as effective as once believed. Always report aggressive bear encounters to the park rangers.

Elk, moose, and bison can also be unpredictable, particularly when young are present, but are not usually dangerous unless approached. Give them a wide berth and wait for them to move off the trail.

Miscellaneous Hazards

- Poison ivy, oak, and sumac should not be a problem on the trails in this book. However, even if you go off-trail and encounter these plants, dealing with the resulting rash is not difficult. You should simply wash the affected area and apply calamine lotion.

- Mosquitoes, black flies, and ticks can be annoying pests on certain hikes and at certain times of the year. You can deter mosquitoes and flies by wearing insect repellants containing deet. For extreme situations I cover up as much as possible and use 100% deet. I have encountered some problems with ticks, particularly in the Rocky Mountain West. After hiking in tick country, especially after hiking off-trail, check for ticks, remove them, and toss them aside. If they have attached to your skin, remove them with tweezers.

- For hikes where the sun is intense, especially at high altitude, cover up as much as possible and use high SPF sunscreen.

- Be careful at overlooks. Edges can be loose, and a gust of wind can send you over the edge. When I was hiking the Precipice Trail to Ocean Path, a hiker fell to his death down the ocean cliffs. Most falls at overlooks can be attributed to carelessness.

- Be watchful for quicksand, particularly on the hike to Keet Seel and in the Zion Narrows. Quicksand forms downstream of boulders and where springs well up. Unlike the Hollywood variety, quicksand on these trails will not suck you under, but it can be alarming, and you might possibly loose a shoe. Watch out for it, and if you feel the sand sink beneath your foot, fall flat and crawl.

- Carry a flashlight or headlamp. Sometimes a hike does not go according to plan, and you can be delayed by any number of circumstances. There have been times when I was very glad I packed a headlamp, and there have been other times when I wish I had. If darkness closes in when you are several miles from the trailhead and you have no light, be assured that the night ahead will be exceedingly uncomfortable.

- For minor hazards, carry a few essentials such as Band-Aids, antibiotic ointment, acetaminophen or ibuprofen, and an Ace bandage.

- Avoid hiking alone, especially on the longer hikes in this book. Hike in a group if possible and don't get separated.

CONDITIONING FOR THE HIKE

The strenuous, and especially the very strenuous, hikes in this book are physically demanding. These hikes require planning and serious preparation. Very strenuous hikes include the Knife Edge of Mount Katahdin, Telescope Peak Trail, Half Dome, Amphitheater Lake–Teton Glacier Trail, Longs Peak Trail, Chicago Basin, Roan Mountain, Keet Seel, Grand Canyon of the Yellowstone Loop, Zion Narrows, Kalalau Trail, Cascade Pass–Sahale Arm Trail, and Chilkoot Trail. When attempting one of these hikes, I begin training about five months in advance. I prepare by walking whenever possible during the week. I also take a long weekend hike, gradually increasing the length up to about 13 miles. Sometimes I will load a pack and walk up and down hills. I have also found that bike riding helps considerably to strengthen my legs. For the Chilkoot Trail hike, I was unable to walk for long distances because of an ankle problem, so I trained exclusively by taking long bike rides up to 100 miles. I found the results to be very satisfactory.

Training is much more important for me now that I am older. There was a time when I could have done most of these hikes with little preparation, but those days are long gone. Even for those who are young and fairly fit, strenuous hikes will be much more enjoyable if you are fully prepared for the physical challenge. I have seen many hikers run completely out of gas several miles from the trailhead—a serious and sometimes dangerous situation.

TRAIL ETIQUETTE

The magnificent trails of America will remain national treasures for our children and grandchildren only if we take care of them and follow a few simple rules of etiquette:

- Always treat the trails, wildlife, fellow hikers, and surrounding landscape with respect.

- Leave only footprints and take only pictures. Stay on the existing trail. Shortcutting switchbacks scars the land, saves little time, and wastes energy. Always pack out what you pack in.

No one likes to see trash that someone else has left behind. Burying trash only leaves the junk for future generations.

- Be courteous to other hikers, bikers, and equestrians on the trail. I am not a great fan of mountain biking or horseback riding on trails, but they have as much right to be there as you do. Move off the trail for bikers and equestrians. Do not pass horses on the trail—they have right of way. When meeting hikers on a narrow trail, uphill traffic normally has right of way.

- Observe animals from a distance. If an animal is on the trail, wait for it to move off. Do not leave the trail to approach an animal for a picture or any other reason. A surprised or irritated animal can be dangerous to you, to others, and to itself.

- Bury human waste in a hole at least 3 inches deep and at least 200 feet away from trails and water sources. This is the one good reason to walk off-trail. Carry a small trowel for this purpose.

- Open fires are no longer considered good practice and will not be necessary for the day hikes in this book. If you find it necessary to heat water or cook, use a small backpacker stove.

- Always observe local rules for the trail or park you are visiting. Ask about current trail conditions and respect any trail closures. Obtain permits if necessary. Sign trail registers when provided at the trailhead, and remember to sign out when you return.

- If dogs are permitted on the trail, always keep them leashed to avoid interaction with animals, hikers, and other dogs. Obey all regulations. National parks, in particular, have strict regulations against pets on trails.

TIPS FOR ENJOYING THE TRAIL

It is likely you will travel a long way to hike the trails in this book and make a considerable investment of both time and money. The following tips will help you enjoy the experience and make the memory a pleasant one:

- Before you go call the park or visit their Web site to determine trail conditions, road closures, or other relevant activities.

- Schedule enough time to enjoy the trail and all it has to offer. Pace yourself. I hiked too fast on many of the hikes in this book. Schedule at least one hour for every 2 miles of trail, plus one hour for every 1,000 feet of elevation gained.

- Plan ahead. Carry all the necessary supplies for the hike, including water, food, sunscreen, insect repellant, first-aid items, clothing, raingear, compass, and flashlight or head-lamp.

- Prepare your body. Read the section on Conditioning for the Hike on page 15 and take it to heart. Nothing can ruin a hike more than pain and exhaustion.

- It's not always possible to be completely flexible when scheduling a hike, but try to adapt your schedule to best advantage. On trails that are likely to be crowded, hike during the week and avoid traditional holidays. Avoid insect seasons when possible, especially black fly season in northern New England. Check the weather forecast and avoid hiking during storms, especially on high mountains and in slot canyons.

- No one is too young to enjoy a hike. However, when hiking with children be mindful of their special requirements. Use common sense to judge a child's abilities and be prepared to carry them when needed. A whining, over-tired child will spoil the hike for everyone.

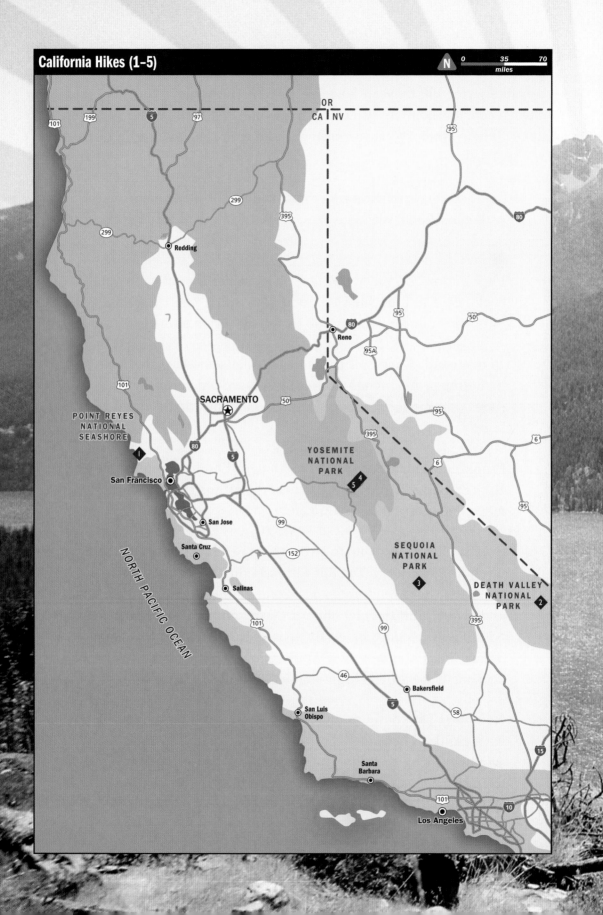

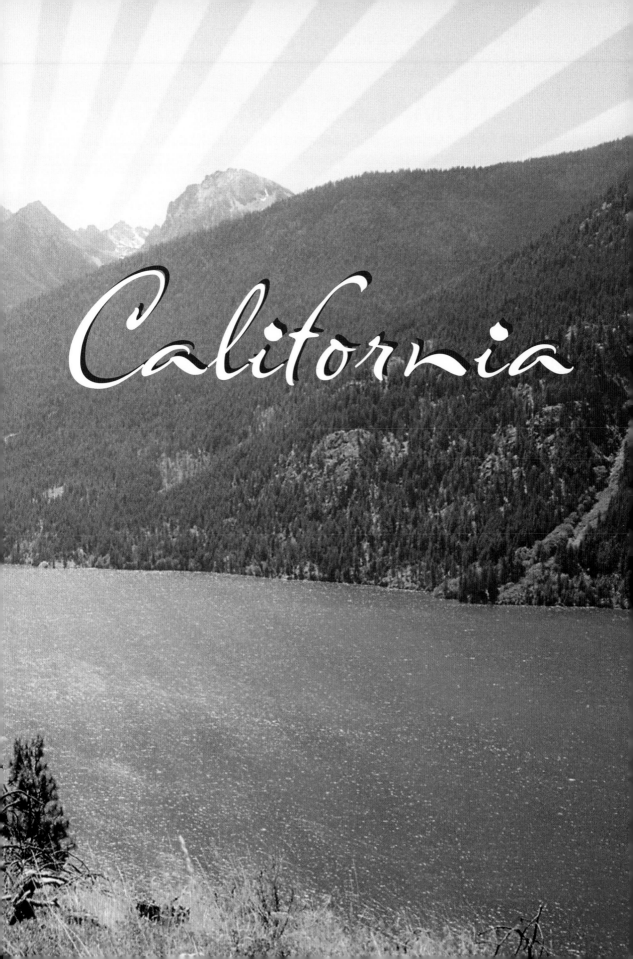

01 TOMALES POINT TRAIL

Location: *Point Reyes National Seashore, CA*
Distance: *9.6 miles*
Elevation Extremes: *125 to 548 feet*
Total Elevation Gain: *1,370 feet*
Difficulty: *Moderate*
USGS Maps: *Tomales 7.5-minute*
Trailhead Coordinates: *N 38° 11' 23.4" W 122° 57' 19.4"*
UTM 10S 0503730 4226930 [WGS84]

EARTHQUAKES AND ELK

They suddenly appeared out of the late evening fog like ghosts from the past. A few tule elk looked down at me from a rise above the trail. Then a few appeared around a bend, while 30 or 40 more grazed peacefully on the grass surrounding Pierce Point Ranch. If not for one of the greatest comeback stories in American history, these elk might not have been here. For thousands of years, as many as 500,000 tule elk thrived in California, but following the Gold Rush of 1849, they were thoughtlessly hunted to the brink of extinction. By 1874 not a single tule elk had been seen for four years until surprised ranch workers discovered a few elk while preparing fields. Fortunately, the landowner felt inclined to protect them, and today their population has recovered to about 3,000 animals. In 1978, ten elk were moved to Tomales Point. Today that same group has surpassed 500 animals to become one of the largest herds in the state. Their appearance was the finale of a truly remarkable California coast hike.

I arrived at the trailhead feeling very lucky for my Tomales Point hike on a late afternoon in May. Like most northern California–coast hikes, fog and wind can make this hike unpleasant almost any time of year. But this day the weather was perfect, and I set off on the trail after a brief look around the historic Pierce Point Ranch. The trail first led west, and after only 20 minutes I was walking atop the spectacular cliffs that rise high above the pounding Pacific surf.

The trail gained 170 feet in elevation to a high prominence overlooking the restless ocean on the left and tranquil Tomales Bay on the right. I looked back toward Drakes Estero, into which Sir Frances Drake allegedly maneuvered his ship in order to make repairs in 1579.

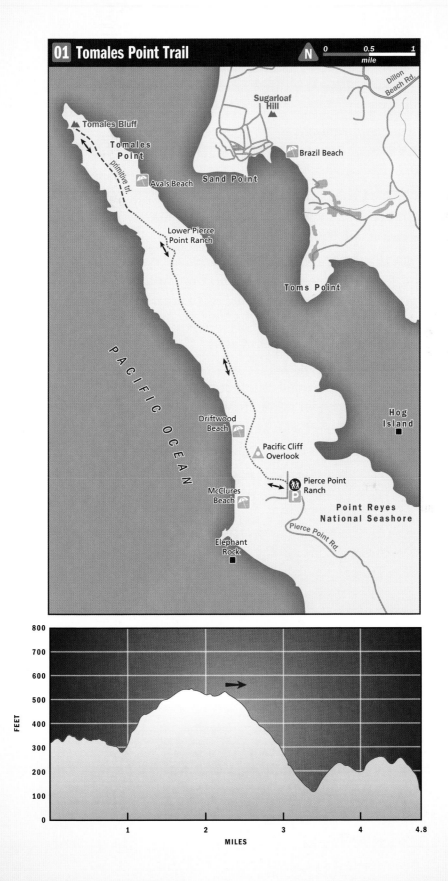

One of his men noted that this landscape was "farre different from the shore, a goodly country . . . stored with many blessings fit for the use of man." Other explorers, sailing past the point in the year 1800, saw large herds of elk roaming the open grasslands. Just 70 years later the elk were gone and thought to be extinct.

The trail meandered along the ridge crest for 1.5 miles with spectacular views in all directions. There are almost no trees on Tomales Point to obstruct the panorama, only fertile waving grassland strewn with an abundance of wildflowers. Here the remarkable topography fully revealed itself. The infamous San Andreas Fault slashes along the western edge of San Francisco, crosses the Golden Gate, and then follows the western edge of the Marin Peninsula. A few miles north, at Point Reyes National Seashore, the fault leaves the California coast, taking Tomales Point with it into the Pacific Ocean. During the great San Francisco earthquake of 1906 alone, Tomales Point slid 20 feet northwestward into the sea!

The trail then descended 140 feet to the Lower Pierce Point Ranch site. Only a few trees now mark the location of the old dairy ranch. Until this point, the trail was in good condition, and I easily walked 3 miles to the lower ranch in an hour and ten minutes.

Pacific Cliff Overlook and Pacific Ocean

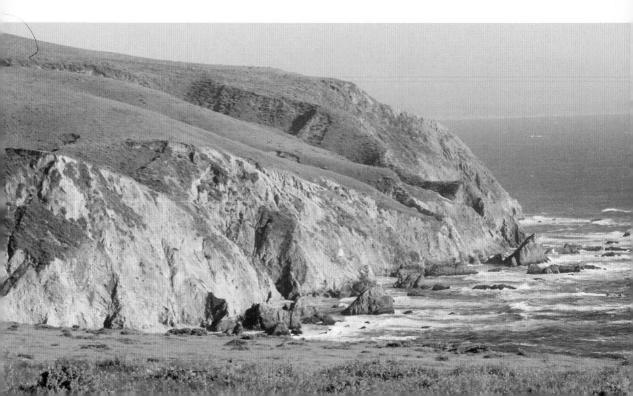

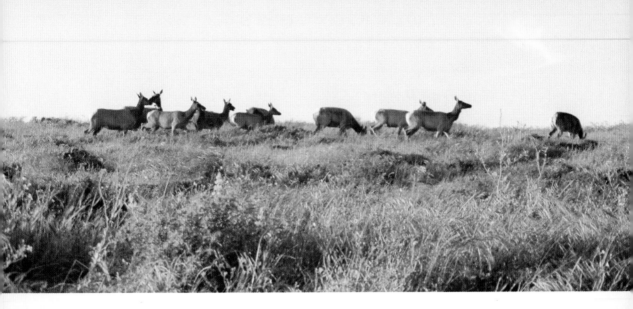

Tule elk appear near dusk.

From the lower ranch, the trail climbed 250 feet to another prominence for more glorious views of the cliffs and Pacific surf. Then the character of the trail abruptly changed from a waving grassland to an unexpected sandy scrub. Loose sand underfoot made walking difficult and tiring as giant thistles and prickly pear took over the landscape. Anyone who chose to wear shorts this far would surely regret the decision. The trail became hard to follow, given the array of elk tracks and bush lupine crowding the paths. I looked ahead, trying to decide if pressing on was worth the effort. The trail descended through sand and scrub to what looked like an anticlimactic end. But I had come this far, so I pushed on. Finally I stepped on the end of the trail, drew a deep breath, and stepped back. The edge looked to be crumbling and unstable, but I was glad I had persisted to the end of the trail. A spectacular cliff in stunning shades of red, orange, and yellow dropped straight down into the sea like a gaping wound. The spectacle was worth the effort it took to get there. It had taken me 1 hour and 40 minutes to hike the full 4.8 miles from Pierce Point Ranch.

The scene was compelling, but the hour was late and I had to get back to the trailhead before nightfall. The return trip proved to be even lovelier as the waning light painted the cliffs and hills soft shades of green and gray. As dusk descended, fog settled in the hollows as I left the coast for the last time. It was 8 p.m. when I finally reached the trailhead at Pierce Point Ranch in gathering darkness. My encounter with the tule elk on the return made a fitting finale for this unforgettable California coast hike.

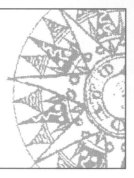

Key Trail Points

From the trailhead at Pierce Point Ranch:
0.9 miles to Pacific cliff overlook
3.2 miles to Lower Pierce Point Ranch
3.8 miles to primitive sandy trail
4.8 miles to Tomales Point cliff
9.6 miles to return to trailhead

DIRECTIONS TO TRAILHEAD AND TRAIL ROUTE

To reach the Tomales Point Trailhead, take US Highway 101 north from the Golden Gate, and then California Highway 1 north for 27 miles along the coast toward Point Reyes National Seashore. Turn west onto Sir Francis Drake Boulevard, and then right onto Pierce Point Road. Finally drive north about 9 miles to the Tomales Point Trailhead at Pierce Point Ranch. There are no entrance or parking fees, and water and toilets are not available.

The trail begins as a broad, double-track road leading west from Pierce Point Ranch. The trail is open to both hikers and equestrians. After about 1 mile the smooth Tomales Point Trail turns north and descends to Windy Gap. The trail then ascends to the ridgeline for sweeping views of the Pacific Ocean on the left and Tomales Bay on the right. The site of the Lower Pierce Point Ranch, now marked only by a few cypress and eucalyptus trees, is reached after 3.2 miles. Beyond the lower ranch, the trail is largely unmaintained, but can be followed through the sand and brush by sticking mainly to the ridgeline. The cliffs at Tomales Point mark the end of the hike, although a faint path continues on down to the tip of the point.

WEATHER AND WILDLIFE

The hike to Tomales Point is especially beautiful from February through May when wildflowers are in abundance, although the days in early winter can also be mild and pleasant. July and August can be

*Cliffs at Tomales Point and
the end of the trail*

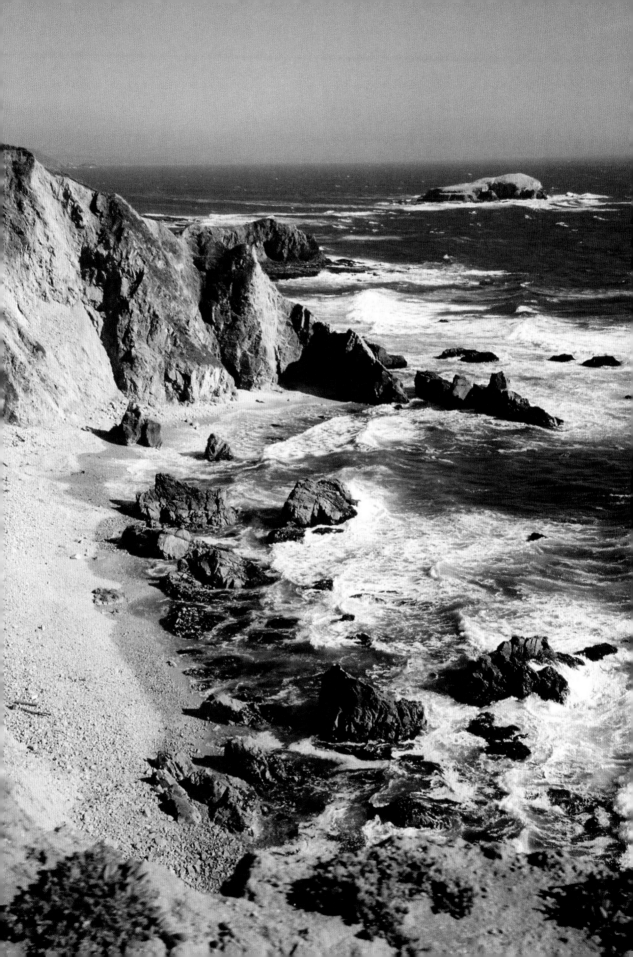

cold, when fog and wind commonly blow in from the Pacific. Strong wind is a common feature of Tomales Point any time of year. Peak flower blooms occur April through May.

A variety of wildlife can be seen on Tomales Point, including rare white deer, seals, sea lions, and more than 300 species of birds. From January to April, impressive gray whales travel past on their annual migration.

Thanks to the success of the tule elk, Tomales Point is also an area within the National Seashore where mountain lions are still seen on a regular basis. The elk rut runs from late July through October, and park volunteers are usually stationed at the trailhead during those weekends to interact with visitors. During the rut, hikers enjoy the special treats of bull elks bugling, rounding up harems of females, and occasionally sparring for supremacy.

The open pastures and cool, moist climate of Tomales Point provide near-ideal conditions for raising dairy cows, and this was the site of one of the earliest and largest industrial-type dairy farms in the state of California. The remains of Pierce Point Ranch at the trailhead and Lower Pierce Point Ranch along the way add historical interest to the hike.

LODGING AND CAMPING

Additional facilities, activities, and information are available at the Bear Valley Visitor Center nearby. There is no overnight lodging in the park, but nearby Inverness offers a few motels and several charming inns and bed-and-breakfasts. Visit **www.pointreyes.org/inverness_marin_county.html** for more information. There are several walk-in campgrounds in the park, with a camp fee of $15 per site.

FEES AND CONTACTS

No entrance fees are required for Point Reyes National Seashore, and pets are not permitted on trails. Visitor information services can be reached at (415) 464-5100, or visit the park Web site at **www.nps.gov/pore** for more information.

02 TELESCOPE PEAK TRAIL

Location: *Death Valley National Park, CA*
Distance: *14.4 miles (16.2 miles without a four-wheel-drive vehicle)*
Elevation Extremes: *8,133 to 11,049 feet*
Total Elevation Gain: *3,250 feet*
Difficulty: *Strenuous*
USGS Maps: *Telescope Peak 7.5-minute*
Trailhead Coordinates: *N 36° 13' 59.4" W 117° 4' 0"*
UTM 11S 0494004 4009817 [WGS84]

WHERE YOU CAN SEE FOREVER

Tom Budlong knocked on our door at the Panamint Springs Resort early one June morning. Tom was an old friend, and a recognized expert on the mountains of southeastern California. When I asked him to nominate a classic American hike, he didn't hesitate. "I'll show you a place where you can see forever—Telescope Peak!" And he delivered. From the airy summit of Telescope Peak, we could look 80 miles east to Charleston Peak above Las Vegas. In the distance to the west are the snowy ramparts of the Sierra Nevada Mountains and the 14,494-foot summit of Mount Whitney, the highest point in the contiguous United States. Directly below is one of the most forbidding and contemptuous places in America—Death Valley. Because of extensive faulting in the valley, this vertical rise from Badwater at minus 282 feet to the 11,049-foot summit of Telescope Peak is one of the greatest in the United States.

Not long after Tom picked me up, we were on our way up Wildrose Canyon on the east side of Death Valley National Park. After a few miles we came upon ten massive beehive-shaped structures built by Chinese laborers in 1876 that looked almost new due to their isolated location and short service life. The Wildrose Charcoal Kilns were used for about three years to process wood into charcoal for the Murdoc Mine smelter located 25 miles to the west. These are one of several boom-and-bust relics of the Death Valley mining era, which lasted about 50 years around the turn of the 20th century. In most cases, the amount of money invested in the mining process far exceeded the value of the ore itself.

Beyond the charcoal kilns the road deteriorated, and I was glad to be riding in Tom's four-wheel-drive Toyota. We arrived at the Mahogany Flat Campground, found the trailhead, and started up toward Telescope

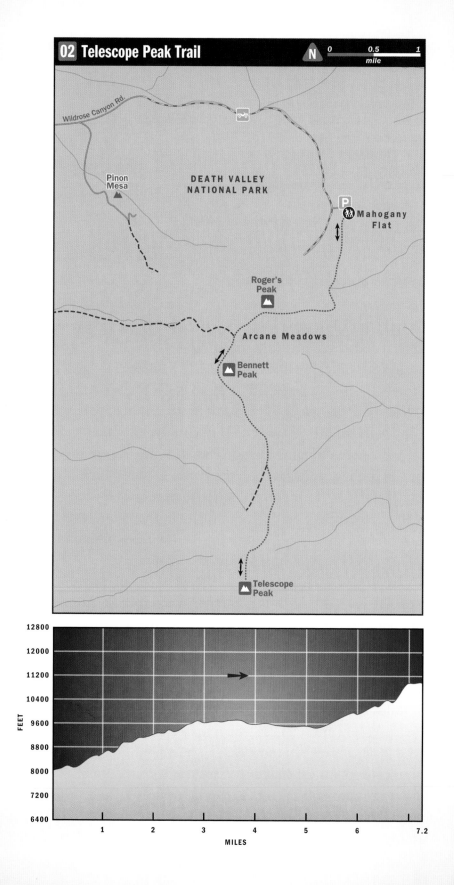

Peak at 9 a.m. Breaks in the juniper and mountain mahogany revealed vistas to the saltpan below, already stewing in the scorching summer heat. Climate and geography combine to make Death Valley one of the driest and hottest places in the world. Only one temperature recording, a 136°F reading in the Sahara Desert, has ever exceeded the 134°F recorded in Death Valley. The valley averages only 1.9 inches of rainfall per year, but its potential evaporation rate is about 150 inches per year. Here, however, 8,000 feet above the valley floor, it was cool and comfortable. We seemed a world away from the oppressive landscape below.

We climbed steadily through clusters of lupine and Indian paintbrush to arrive at Arcane Meadows at 10 a.m. From Arcane Meadows the trail contoured along the west side of Bennett Peak, and we rested in the shade of some twisted pines. Arcane Meadows and Bennett Peak were named for the Arcane and Bennett parties who were trapped in Death Valley in 1849. These unfortunate families were part of a huge tide of prospectors rushing toward the newly discovered gold fields of California. A few of the '49ers left their wagon train to take a shortcut. This "shortcut" led them down into one of the most barren and unfor-

giving places in America. Once in the valley, a towering mountain range and dead-end canyons blocked escape to the west. The unlucky '49ers split into groups, and most managed to escape with their lives and animals—all except the Bennett and Arcane parties. Too weak to move, they stayed in their desolate camp until rescued several weeks later.

The trail descended slightly to a pass between Bennett Peak and Telescope Peak, where we began a long series of switchbacks up through

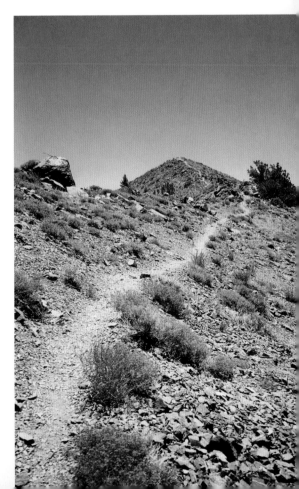

Trail to the summit of
Telescope Peak

limber and bristlecone pine forest. The bristlecone pines on Telescope Peak appear to be nearly as old as those in the celebrated Methuselah Grove of ancient pines, perhaps over 4,000 years old, but have not yet been dated. These gnarled trees have perfected the art of survival in a land that appears completely inhospitable in nearly every respect.

Finally the summit appeared beyond a sharp and airy ridge, a fitting climax to a wonderful hike. The walk along the ridge was exhilarating, as was the summit itself, which rises head and shoulders above any of its neighbors. Only from this unique place can one see both the high and low points of the 48 contiguous states from a single viewpoint. Thousands of feet below, Badwater and Dantes View were shimmering in 115°F midday heat. The climb had taken us three-and-a-half hours, and we paused for a well-deserved lunch with a view.

After lunch we retraced our steps back to the Mahogany Flat Trailhead in a little over three hours, arriving back at the trailhead at 4:20 p.m., tired but elated. In addition to one of the most unique and beautiful mountain vistas in the world, Telescope Peak had given me a whole new perspective on the austere and unforgiving Death Valley.

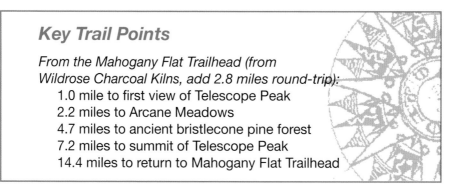

Key Trail Points

From the Mahogany Flat Trailhead (from Wildrose Charcoal Kilns, add 2.8 miles round-trip):
   1.0 mile to first view of Telescope Peak
   2.2 miles to Arcane Meadows
   4.7 miles to ancient bristlecone pine forest
   7.2 miles to summit of Telescope Peak
   14.4 miles to return to Mahogany Flat Trailhead

DIRECTIONS TO TRAILHEAD AND TRAIL ROUTE

Telescope Peak Trailhead is located at the Mahogany Flat Campground past the Wildrose Charcoal Kilns. To reach the campground and trailhead, turn south from California State Route 190 at Emigrant, and drive 21 miles south on Emigrant Canyon Road. Then turn left (east) and travel 7 miles up Wildrose Canyon Road to the Wildrose Charcoal Kilns and Wildrose Campground. The road above the charcoal kilns to Mahogany Flat Campground climbs about 1,200 feet in 1.4 miles, and is suitable only for high-clearance, preferably four-wheel-drive vehicles. If this road cannot be driven, then add 1,200 feet elevation gain and 2.8

miles round-trip distance to the already strenuous hike from Mahogany Flat. An easier alternative might be to pack up and overnight at the campground, and then attempt the hike the next day. But all water must be carried up from Wildrose, since there is no water available at either the campground or on the hike.

Telescope Peak Trail begins at an elevation of 8,133 feet at the south end of the campground in dense juniper and mountain mahogany and climbs steadily around the east flank of Rogers Peak to Arcane Meadows at 9,600 feet. From the meadows the trail contours west, then slightly down to a pass between Bennett Peak and Telescope Peak. From this pass at about 9,500 feet, the trail switchbacks up through ancient bristlecone and limber pine to the Telescope Peak summit at 11,049 feet. The prominent summit offers spectacular vistas, and is the only place where one can see both Badwater and Mount Whitney from a single viewpoint. As described by one pioneer, "You can see so far, it's just like looking through a telescope."

Return to the Mahogany Flat Campground Trailhead, or to the Wildrose Charcoal Kilns, by the same route in reverse.

Wildflowers in Arcane Meadow

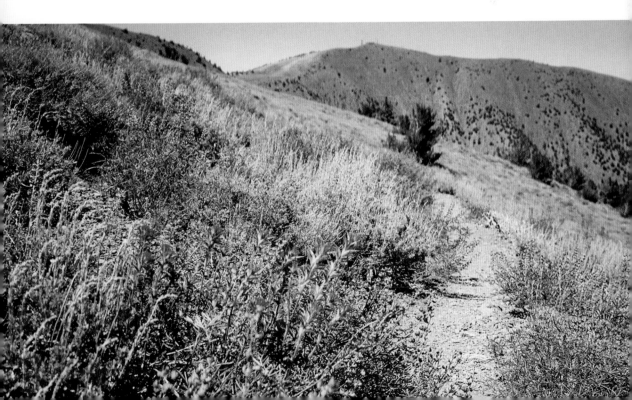

WEATHER AND WILDLIFE

Only a few tourists choose to experience firsthand the blistering summer heat of Death Valley from June to August. When traveling through Death Valley in the summer, the sun burns a savage warning to the unwary. Check your vehicle gauges frequently, and if your car breaks down, stay with it. Even in the 21st century, people die from the heat in this harsh environment. Winter is the heavy tourist season for Death Valley, but not a good time to hike Telescope Peak. Hikers in winter should be prepared for deep snow, should have crampons and ice axes, and know how to use them. Deep winter snow on Telescope Peak can last into May and sometimes even into early June.

Animals most commonly seen in the valley include coyotes, roadrunners, ground squirrels, and lizards. Lucky hikers may catch sight of bighorn sheep high on Telescope Peak.

LODGING AND CAMPING

Lodging within the park can be found at Stovepipe Wells Village (**www.stovepipewells.com**), Furnace Creek Inn and Ranch Resort (**www.furnacecreekresort.com**), and Panamint Springs Resort (**www.deathvalley.com/psr**).

Campgrounds convenient to Telescope Peak include Wildrose and Mahogany Flat. Both of these campgrounds are free, but only Wildrose has water available. Mahogany Flat Campground is open only from March through November. The main full-service campground in the park is Furnace Creek, located near the Furnace Creek Visitor Center. Furnace Creek Campground is open year-round, has 136 sites, and accepts reservations. Fees vary from $18 per night during the winter to $12 per night in summer.

FEES AND CONTACTS

The entrance fee for Death Valley is $20 per vehicle for a seven-day pass. For more information, contact Death Valley National Park, PO Box 579, Death Valley, CA 92328-0570, or call the park at (760) 786-3200. For information on the Internet, visit **www.nps.gov/deva.**

View of Badwater from
Telescope Peak

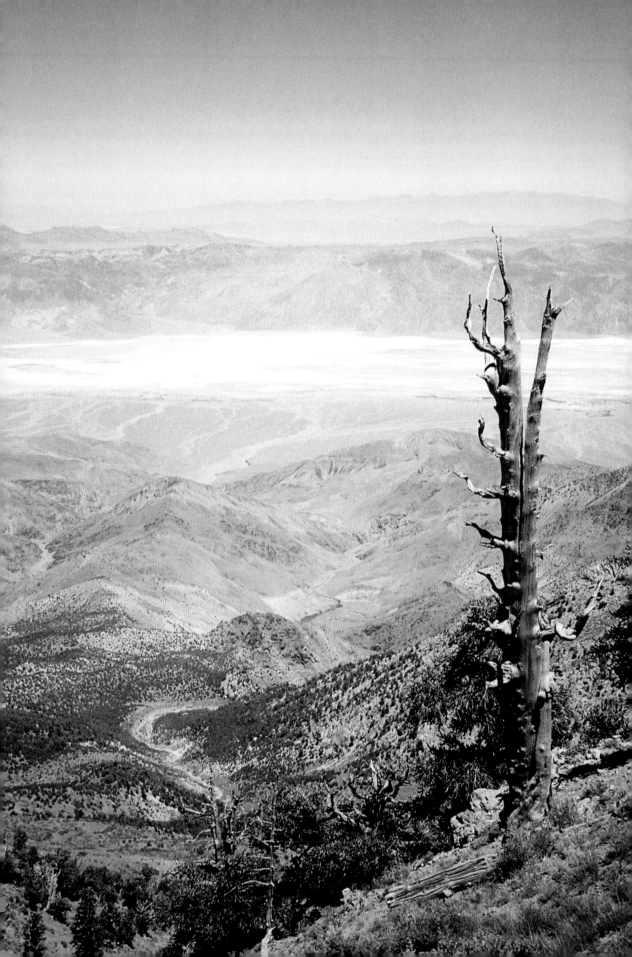

03 GIANT FOREST
(TRAIL OF THE SEQUOIAS, CONGRESS, AND ALTA TRAILS)

Location: *Sequoia National Park, CA*
Distance: *8.5 miles*
Elevation Extremes: *6,560 to 7,320 feet*
Total Elevation Gain: *1,250 feet*
Difficulty: *Moderate*
USGS Maps: *Giant Forest 15-minute, Lodgepole 15-minute*
Trailhead Coordinates: *N 36° 34' 49.8" W 118° 45' 3.6"*
UTM 0343340 4049770 [WGS84]

AT THE FEET OF GIANTS

I was shocked as the acrid smoke burned our eyes and offended our lungs. Our trail did not enter the controlled burn area, but ran alongside it for several hundred yards. The canopy of the forest was not involved, but many trees, including giant sequoias, were fully ablaze 20 to 30 feet above the ground. Park service personnel were nowhere to be seen. Suddenly, somewhere in the burn there was a gigantic crash as a tree toppled to the forest floor. Is this the way a "controlled" burn is supposed to be? I have no training in forest management, and have never seen a controlled burn up close before, but what I was seeing didn't look very controlled to me. It was alarming! I could only assume that those conducting the burn knew what they were doing and were fully aware of what was happening.

On the day before our early-summertime hike, I had a sinking feeling as we turned west on California Highway 198 toward Sequoia National Park. A gigantic plume of smoke rose into the clear California sky, and it appeared to be coming directly from the park. I had planned an extraordinary hike at the feet of giants—including four of the five largest living things on the planet, a cabin constructed inside a hollowed-out sequoia log, and ancient bedrock mortars used by prehistoric peoples. Now our hike seemed very much in jeopardy.

Upon arriving in the park, I also learned that the Congress Trail, where I planned to begin our hike, was undergoing maintenance and was closed to hikers. But after talking with park rangers and brooding over trail maps, I determined that we could still do 80 percent of the route I intended by starting at the Crescent Meadow parking area. The

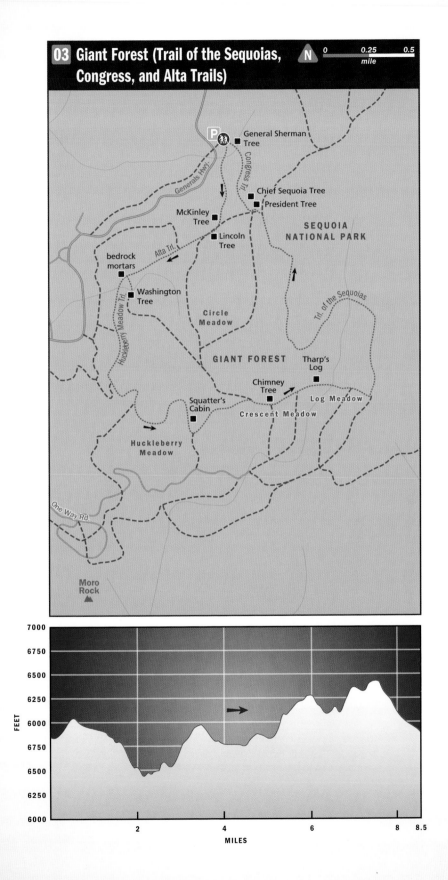

03 Giant Forest (Trail of the Sequoias, Congress, and Alta Trails)

N

0   0.25   0.5
mile

General Sherman Tree

Congress Trl.

Generals Hwy.

Chief Sequoia Tree

President Tree

McKinley Tree

SEQUOIA NATIONAL PARK

Alta Trl.

Lincoln Tree

bedrock mortars

Huckleberry Meadow Trl.

Washington Tree

Circle Meadow

Trl. of the Sequoias

GIANT FOREST

Tharp's Log

Chimney Tree

Log Meadow

Squatter's Cabin

Crescent Meadow

Huckleberry Meadow

One Way Rd.

Moro Rock

Elevation Profile

FEET				
7000				
6750				
6500				
6250				
6000				
6750				
6500				
6250				
6000				

2   4   6   8   8.5

MILES

35

order of the hike would be altered, but we could still take in nearly all of the noteworthy features of this extraordinary forest.

I met my old friend Tom Budlong the next morning for breakfast at Stony Creek Lodge. It was late June, and the weather was perfect. After driving to the Crescent Meadow parking area, we started down the trail at 9:30 a.m. Crescent Meadow was one of four meadows that we would pass by on this hike. These meadows are too wet to support sequoia growth, but are filled with sedges and wildflowers in midsummer. However, the meadows also serve another purpose. Only from a meadow can the full profile of the giant sequoias be seen and fully grasped. John Muir later called Crescent Meadow in particular the "Gem of the Sierra."

At the end of the meadow was the spectacular Chimney Tree. Fire-hollowed by natural fires over hundreds of years, it did not finally succumb until ravaged by a careless campfire 60 years ago. I have heard it said that only toppling kills giant sequoias and that fire cannot harm them. But the Chimney Tree, as well as other examples along the trail, confirmed that fire can also kill these giants.

Crescent Meadow in Seqouia National Park

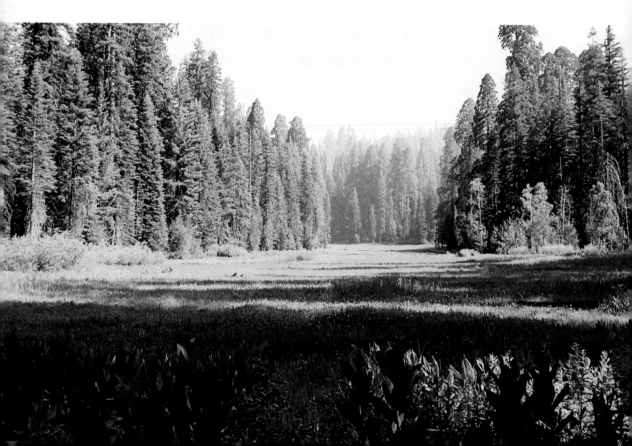

Soon after turning right onto the Trail of the Sequoias, we arrived at Tharp's Log on the fringe of Log Meadow at 10 a.m. Here we took a few minutes to rest and to study the cabin constructed inside a colossal sequoia log, where pioneer cattleman Hale Tharp established a residence to lay claim to this tract of land. The cabin was large enough to be comfortable, but looked rather like the home of a hobbit or an elf. The giant trees surrounding us seemed to magnify this effect by shifting our perspective. John Muir later called this cabin "a noble den." What a delight it must have been to actually live at the feet of these gentle giants.

We surmounted a ridge, then continued north above Crescent Creek. We were near the eastern edge of the grove, but still marveled at the imposing stands of giant trees. After crossing Crescent Creek, we mounted another ridge to the highest point of the trail, and then descended to meet Congress Trail at the Chief Sequoia Tree and the enormous President Tree at 11 a.m. Congress Trail was closed, but we could bypass it on Alta Trail, passing by the McKinley Tree and later on the Lincoln Tree. Here within the Giant Forest grow the largest living things on the face of the earth. There are 75 known groves of giant sequoias in the high sierra, but no other grove manifests the beauty or awesome impact of the Giant Forest. This location, with its gentle, well-watered terrain and mild winter climate, represents the optimum site for giant sequoia growth.

A short spur took us up a knoll to the Washington Tree, the second largest tree on earth. Although a little smaller than the General Sherman Tree, the Washington Tree, standing alone on top of the knoll, seemed all the more noble and invincible. Just below the Washington Tree was a grove of small sequoias—born of fire—that looked like a brood of little children at the feet of a proud parent.

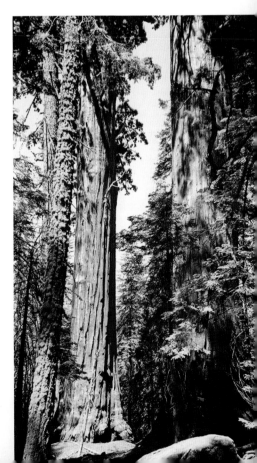

General Sherman Tree—
largest living thing on earth

When prospectors and hunters first explored the central portion of the Sierra Nevada in the early 1850s, they were astonished to find gigantic trees of a distinctive cinnamon color. Early reports were met with doubt. The very idea of a tree with a circumference of over 100 feet seemed preposterous. Skepticism continued for years among those who had not seen sequoias firsthand. Those who saw a section of a giant sequoia taken to Europe for display regarded it as a hoax, and well they might. Although at least one species of tree lives longer, one has a greater diameter, and three grow taller, the giant sequoias stand alone as the largest living things on the planet. The largest giant sequoias are over 300 feet tall, 40 feet in diameter, weigh up to 1,350 tons, and have bark more than 30 inches thick and branches 8 feet in diameter. Each year they add enough wood to make a 60-foot-tall tree of usual proportions. The giant sequoias simply must be seen to be believed. Although shamelessly logged in the late 1890s, the big trees are now protected thanks to the tireless efforts of conservationists like John Muir.

Back on Alta/Huckleberry Meadow Trail, we soon came to the bedrock mortars where early inhabitants ground acorns and pine nuts. The mortars were deep, and must have been fashioned over centuries of use. We paused to wonder what the lives of these Native Americans were like, and what they thought of these towering pillars, the very same ancient trees that we see here today.

Farther along, Huckleberry Meadow Trail ran directly beside the "controlled" burn. We hurried up the ridge to get away from the thick smoke, which was becoming oppressive.

After skirting Huckleberry Meadow and Crescent Meadow, we arrived back at the parking area at 1 p.m. The hike had taken us three-and-a-half hours to complete.

There is no question that this walk through the Giant Forest of Sequoia National Park is one of the great classic hikes of America. The coastal redwoods of California are certainly impressive, and other trees are much older, but these giant sequoias are simply the most amazing trees I have ever seen. Words fail to describe the impact and majesty of these Goliaths. Walking at the feet of these giant trees, with their beautiful cinnamon color, is an almost religious experience, and one never to be forgotten.

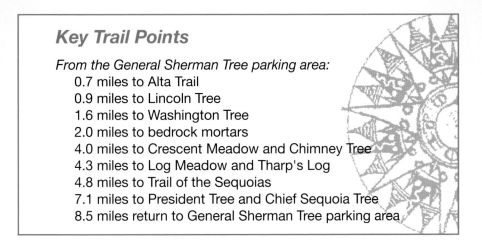

Key Trail Points

From the General Sherman Tree parking area:
- 0.7 miles to Alta Trail
- 0.9 miles to Lincoln Tree
- 1.6 miles to Washington Tree
- 2.0 miles to bedrock mortars
- 4.0 miles to Crescent Meadow and Chimney Tree
- 4.3 miles to Log Meadow and Tharp's Log
- 4.8 miles to Trail of the Sequoias
- 7.1 miles to President Tree and Chief Sequoia Tree
- 8.5 miles return to General Sherman Tree parking area

DIRECTIONS TO TRAILHEAD AND TRAIL ROUTE

Since this magnificent loop uses many trails and has several turns, it is recommended to first stop at the Giant Forest Museum or Lodgepole Visitor Center and purchase a Giant Forest Trail Map for $2. This will minimize the possibility of taking wrong turns and traveling extra miles.

This hike begins at the General Sherman parking area on Generals Highway in Sequoia National Park. General Sherman is recognized as the largest tree in the world, and the parking area and footpaths here are usually crowded. But take a few moments to savor the immensity of this Goliath, whose trunk weighs an estimated 1,385 tons! From the parking area, take Congress Trail 0.7 miles to the intersection of Alta Trail at the McKinley Tree. Turn right on Alta Trail and follow it 0.6 miles to Huckleberry Meadow Trail. Along Alta Trail you will pass by the Lincoln Tree, the fifth-largest tree in the world. At the junction with Huckleberry Meadow Trail, take a short spur 0.3 miles to the left to see the Washington Tree, the second-largest tree in the world. The Washington Tree looks all the more overwhelming in this setting, since people and human developments do not surround it. Return to the junction of Alta and Huckleberry Meadow trails.

Only 0.1 mile farther along Alta and Huckleberry Meadow trails are the bedrock mortars used by early Native Americans to grind acorns and pine nuts that were an important part of their diet. After another 0.5 miles, leave Alta Trail and continue left and uphill on Huckleberry Meadow Trail. Another mile brings you to Squatter's Cabin, one of the oldest remaining structures in Sequoia National Park. Continue left 0.3 miles past Huckleberry Meadow to a junction

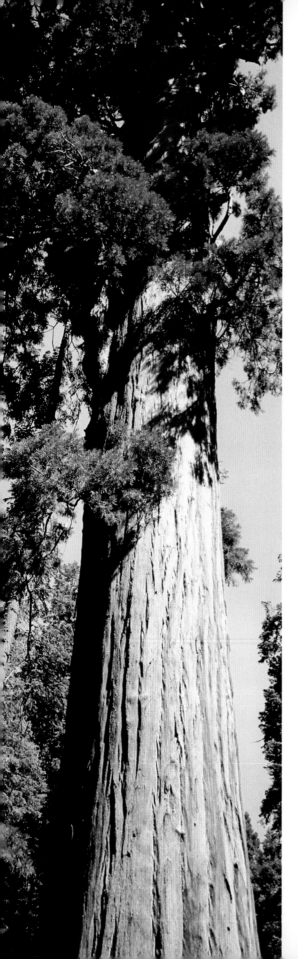

The Washington Tree in the
Giant Forest

with Trail of the Sequoias and turn
right. You will be on Trail of the Sequoias for the next 3.3 miles, passing Crescent Meadow, Chimney
Tree, and Log Meadow to arrive at
Tharp's Log. Take a few moments
at Tharp's Log to rest and examine
this remarkable cabin built inside a
sequoia log.

From Log Meadow, Trail of the
Sequoias climbs uphill and then
winds back through some of the finest stands of giant sequoias, away
from the crowds and along some of
the more scenic parts of the plateau. Trail of the Sequoias rejoins
Congress Trail at the Chief Sequoia
Tree and the President Tree, the
fourth-largest tree in the world.
Follow Congress Trail back to the
General Sherman Tree and the
trailhead at the parking lot.

WEATHER AND WILDLIFE

The Giant Forest in summer generally has warm days and cool nights.
Rain is more common in fall, with
chilly nights. There is generally a
deep blanket of snow in the Giant
Forest from December to May. The
ground in the groves is still snow-
covered through most of spring.

Animals commonly seen in Sequoia National Park include coyotes, black bears, ringtails, and mule deer. Wolverines, badgers, and bighorn sheep are rarer. Black bears are a common problem, and measures must be taken to protect all food and prevent accidental encounters. We saw several bears during our stay in the park.

LODGING AND CAMPING

There are three full-service lodges within Sequoia and Kings Canyon National Parks (see **www.nps.gov/seki/planyourvisit/lodging.htm**). In addition, nearby Stony Creek Lodge, located outside park boundaries, is the closest to the Giant Forest. See **www.sequoia-kingscanyon .com/stonycreeklodge.html** for more information.

The two parks also have 14 campgrounds with a total of 800 campsites. The four campgrounds most convenient to the hike include Lodgepole, Dorst, Buckeye Flat, and Potwisha. Both Lodgepole and Dorst, where campsites are $20 per night, take reservations. Buckeye Flat and Potwisha are both located in the foothills at lower elevations, do not take reservations, and are $18 per site per night.

FEES AND CONTACTS

Sequoia National Park is open 365 days a year, although the Generals Highway is subject to brief closure following winter storms. A seven-day pass for the park, purchased at either of the two entrance stations, is $20 per vehicle. Pets are not permitted on trails.

For more information, visit **www.nps.gov/seki** or phone (559) 565-3341. Or make contact by mail at Sequoia and Kings Canyon National Parks, 47050 Generals Highway, Three Rivers, CA 93271.

Done ✓

04 YOSEMITE FALLS TRAIL

Location: *Yosemite National Park, CA*
Distance: *7.2 miles*
Elevation Extremes: *3,990 to 6,710 feet*
Total Elevation Gain: *3,510 feet*
Difficulty: *Strenuous*
USGS Maps: *Half Dome 7.5-minute, Yosemite Falls 7.5-minute*
Trailhead Coordinates: *N 37° 44' 29.4" W 119° 36' 9"*
                        UTM 11S 0270715 4180310 [WGS84]

TO THE BRINK

At first glance, it seems improbable that a trail could be constructed from the valley floor to the top of Yosemite Falls, given the seemingly impassable cliffs that surround it. But Yosemite Falls Trail is in fact one of the oldest trails in Yosemite National Park, having been built from 1873 to 1877. This remarkable trail features unique views of the upper falls, as well as stunning vistas of the valley below. Yosemite Falls Trail is physically demanding, and the airy path that leads to the very brink of the falls is not for the faint of heart, but the rewards are undeniably worth the effort.

It was hot in the valley in late June, and there was little room on the packed Yosemite Valley shuttle bus. I wistfully recalled my first trip to Yosemite years ago when there was no shuttle bus, and we could drive and park anywhere. Unfortunately, in addition to being the most spectacular valley in America, Yosemite is also one of the most crowded. Packed buses shuttle crowds of visitors from giant central parking lots to attractions and trailheads, and smoke from campfires hang heavy on hot summer nights.

My wife Mary Fran, our 12-year-old daughter Jenny, and I got off the bus at shuttle bus stop 7 near Yosemite Lodge and walked across the street to Sunnyside Campground. Finding Yosemite Falls Trailhead took a few minutes as valley trails seemed to crisscross from every direction. We started up the steep switchbacks at noon.

By 12:30 p.m. we needed a break, and paused for lunch on some rocks along the trail. Jenny was seated high on a rock when her jaw dropped open.

Upper Yosemite Falls from
Yosemite Falls Trail

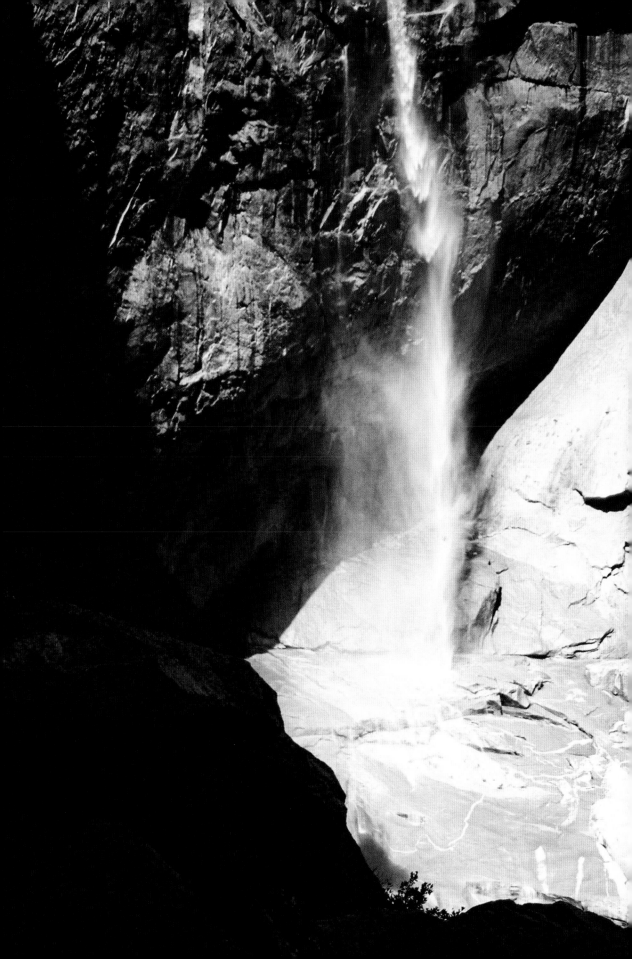

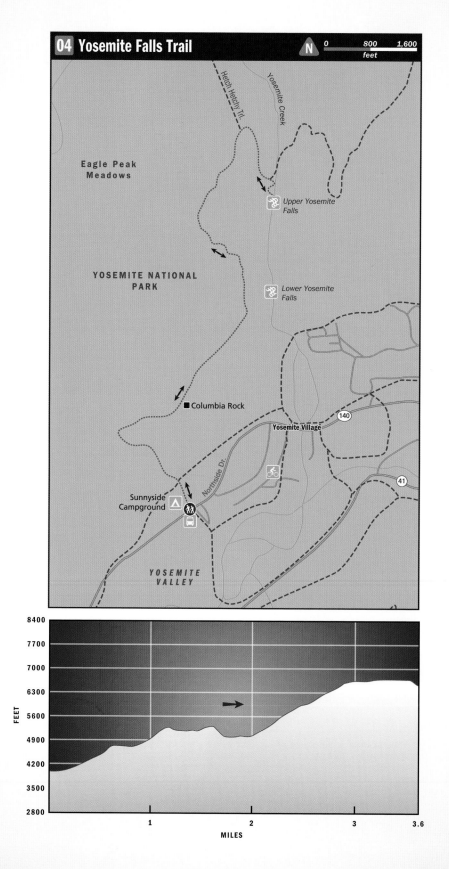

She pointed down the slope and said "Cat . . . big . . . big cat!" There, walking among the boulders about 100 feet downhill, was a bobcat, apparently stalking something and completely unconcerned about our presence. What a surprise! Bobcats are normally nocturnal and not usually seen this close to heavy tourist areas. We watched it for nearly 15 minutes and pointed it out to other excited hikers coming up the trail. It was one of those unexpected, magical moments that make a hike like this truly unforgettable. Soon after lunch Mary Fran and Jenny turned back, leaving me to finish the strenuous hike to the top.

Columbia Rock, about 1,000 feet above the valley floor, provided the first impressive view of Yosemite Valley and a welcome resting place. Yosemite Valley is simply the most spectacular valley in America, and possibly on the face of the earth. Majestic rock skyscrapers tower on all sides, and ribbons of waterfalls plummet from the valley rim. The falls of Yosemite are so high that the water seems to drop from the sky in a slow-motion dance with the wind. Three of the world's ten highest

Swimming pool at the brink of the falls

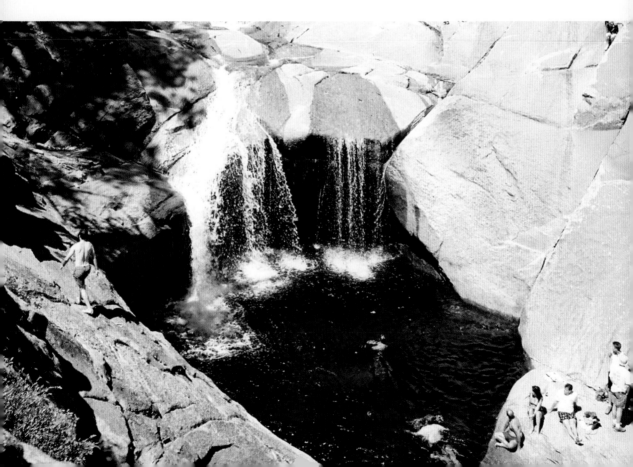

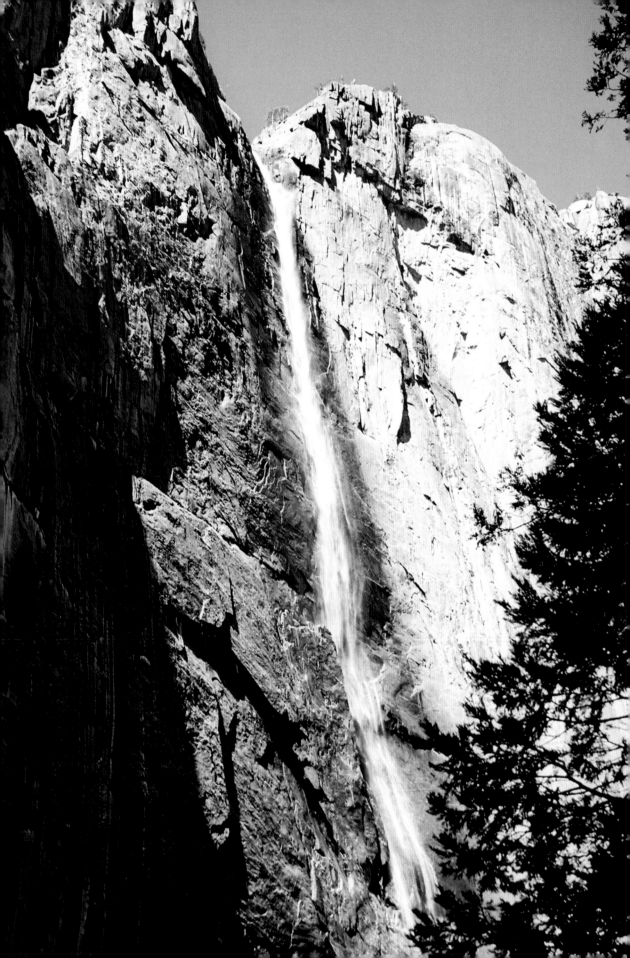

waterfalls are here including the crown jewel of Yosemite, the majestic Yosemite Falls.

From Columbia Rock the trail contoured north on a series of ledges, then descended toward the bottom of the upper falls. The thunder of the falls increased, and the sun played with rainbows in the spray. The fall was so high that some of the water just seemed to disappear and never quite reach the rocks below. This awe-inspiring cascade drops a total of 2,565 feet in three sections from the north wall of the valley. Upper Yosemite Falls, the highest waterfall in North America, plunges a sheer 1,430 feet from the brink of the cliffs above to thunder on the rocks below. I joined a long line of hikers trudging up the switchbacks toward the cliffs above. This trail was definitely not a wilderness experience, but the crowds did not diminish the undeniable beauty and power of the highest waterfall in America.

I reached the top of the switchbacks, turned right toward Yosemite Point at the Hetch Hetchy Trail, then right again toward the top of the falls. Descending the rocks, I found the trail leading down toward Yosemite Creek, and then back again to drop down a steep, narrow stairway with a threadlike handrail. It was a spectacular and unsettling place. Two other hikers were struggling with fear and finally decided to turn back. I descended the stairs to the brink of the falls at 2:40 p.m., and took in the spectacular scene for 20 minutes. Airborne mist was blowing up from the cascade and shimmering in the afternoon sun. Too soon it was time to descend.

The descent was routine until I reached a point about halfway between the bottom of the falls and Columbia Rock. There, lying prone in the middle of the trail, was a man in his mid-30s. At first he looked to be in good health, but closer examination revealed that all his leg muscles had cramped, leaving him helpless. He was unable to stand, let alone walk. "Do you have a banana? Do you have anything with potassium?" he begged. He had no water, and it seemed to me more likely that he was suffering from severe dehydration. I gave him what water I could spare and went on down the trail. He had a cell phone and was about to call for help, and his two companions were ready to provide him with assistance if needed. The south-facing Yosemite Falls Trail can be very hot and dry, and should not be taken lightly on a hot summer day.

Upper Yosemite Falls from Yosemite Falls Trail

I reached Sunnyside Campground at 4:45 p.m., only 1 hour and 45 minutes after leaving the top of the falls, and met Mary Fran and Jenny for a cold drink at Yosemite Lodge. My hike up Yosemite Falls Trail was an unforgettable experience, with rewarding vistas, the feel of spray on my face, rainbows dancing in the mist, and the constant thunder of America's highest falls in my ears.

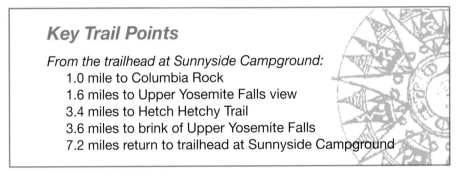

Key Trail Points

From the trailhead at Sunnyside Campground:
- 1.0 mile to Columbia Rock
- 1.6 miles to Upper Yosemite Falls view
- 3.4 miles to Hetch Hetchy Trail
- 3.6 miles to brink of Upper Yosemite Falls
- 7.2 miles return to trailhead at Sunnyside Campground

DIRECTIONS TO TRAILHEAD AND TRAIL ROUTE

Upper Yosemite Falls Trail begins near the kiosk on the west side of the Sunnyside Campground parking area. Parking at Sunnyside is for the campground only, so it is best to take the Yosemite Valley shuttle bus to shuttle bus stop 7. The trail first switchbacks steeply up through boulders and trees to Columbia Rock, 1,000 feet above the valley floor. From Columbia Rock the trail descends slightly along a sequence of ledges to a point directly west of the base of the upper falls. Here hikers begin a series of relentless switchbacks up an old talus slope. But the frequent and ever-changing view of the towering falls makes it easier to accept the effort.

From the top of the switchbacks, the trail leads gently up and over a rocky ridge and then finally down to the top of the falls. As you descend toward the falls, the trail seems to end more than once, but a final exposed stairway with an airy handrail leads to a dramatic ledge at the very brink of the cascade. A few hikers reward themselves with a cold swim in the pools just above the rim of the falls.

Return to the trailhead at Sunnyside Campground by retracing your steps the same route in reverse.

WEATHER AND WILDLIFE

Summer temperatures in the valley may reach 100°F, but nights are usually cool. Yosemite Falls Trail can be hot and unforgiving in summer, and hikers should be sure to carry plenty of water. Yosemite Valley seldom experiences severe weather in winter, and the southern exposure of the trail keeps it relatively free of snow and ice in the off-season.

The most commonly seen mammals in the park include squirrels, coyotes, mule deer, black bears, and marmots. Less often seen are mountain lions, foxes, lynx, and bobcats. Rattlesnakes are common below 9,000 feet, but are seldom seen by visitors. As with most other national parks, pets are not permitted on trails.

LODGING AND CAMPING

Two lodges are available inside the valley, including the Yosemite Lodge and the more luxurious Ahwanee. Lodging reservations can be made by calling (801) 559-4854 or online at **www.yosemitepark.com,** and should be made several months in advance. Many other lodging and service options are located outside the entrance stations.

Six campgrounds are located inside Yosemite Valley, where fees are typically $20 per night. Reservations are recommended for camping in the valley, and can be made four months in advance by calling (877) 444-6777. Some campsites are available on a first-come, first-serve basis, but in summer these typically fill up well before noon.

FEES AND CONTACTS

The entrance fee for Yosemite National Park is $20 per vehicle for a seven-day pass. For more information, write the Superintendent, Yosemite National Park, CA 95389-0577, or call (209) 379-2648. For information on the Internet, visit **www.nps.gov/yose.**

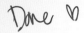

Done ♡

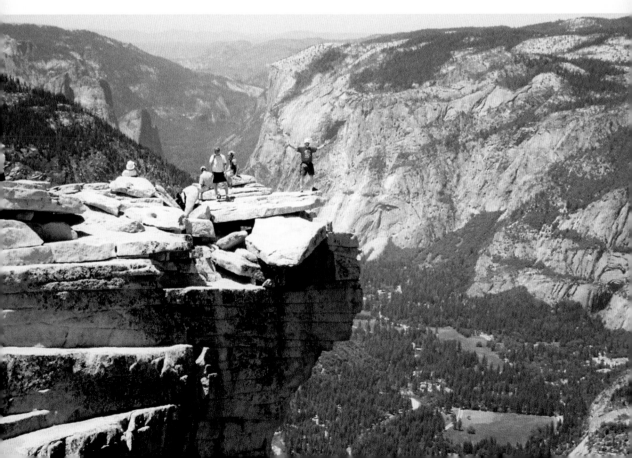

05 HALF DOME

Location: *Yosemite National Park, CA*
Distance: *17.4 miles*
Elevation Extremes: *4,035 to 8,842 feet*
Total elevation Gain: *4,910 feet*
Difficulty: *Very Strenuous*
USGS Maps: *Half Dome 7.5-minute*
Trailhead Coordinates: *N 37° 43' 56.4" W 119° 33' 35.4"*
UTM 11S 0270715 4180310 [WGS84]

STAIRWAY TO HEAVEN

Excitement welled up in me as I stepped off the shuttle bus at stop 16 early on that July morning. This was the California hike I had been waiting for, and I had trained hard for it. Many years had passed since I first climbed Half Dome in my youth, and at 57 years old, I was no longer certain that I was up to the task. I stepped off the first Yosemite

Standing on the "Visor" on top of Half Dome

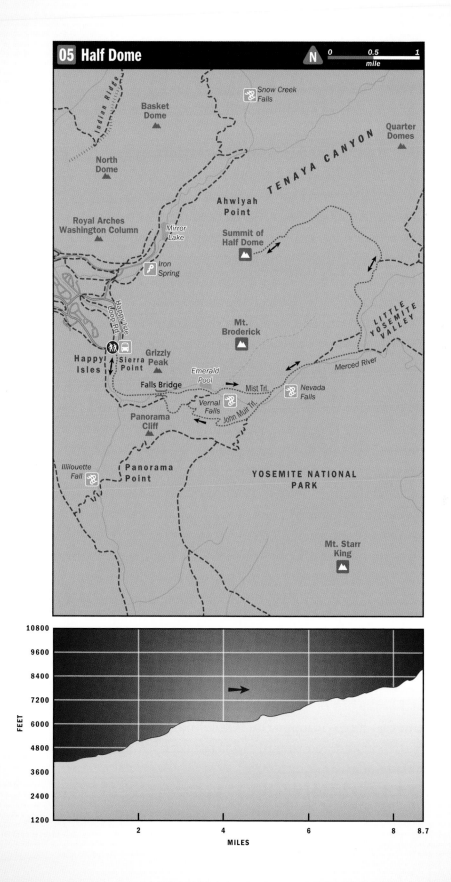

05 Half Dome

N

0   0.5   1
mile

Indian Ridge

Basket Dome ▲

Snow Creek Falls

Quarter Domes ▲

North Dome ▲

TENAYA CANYON

Ahwiyah Point

Royal Arches Washington Column ▲

Mirror Lake

Summit of Half Dome ▲

Iron Spring

LITTLE YOSEMITE VALLEY

Happy Isle Loop Rd.

Mt. Broderick ▲

Merced River

Happy Isles

Sierra Point ▲

Grizzly Peak ▲

Emerald Pool

Mist Trl.

Nevada Falls

Falls Bridge

Vernal Falls

John Muir Trl.

Panorama Cliff ▲

Illilouette Fall

Panorama Point

YOSEMITE NATIONAL PARK

Mt. Starr King ▲

FEET

10800
9600
8400
7200
6000
4800
3600
2400
1200

2   4   6   8   8.7

MILES

Valley shuttle bus of the morning, and started up the trail toward Half Dome at 7:45 a.m.

Half Dome ". . . is a crest of granite . . . perfectly inaccessible, being probably the only one of all the prominent points about the Yosemite which never has been, and never will be, trodden by human foot." With these words, an early California Geological Survey report dismissed the possibility of climbing Half Dome. But only a few years later John Anderson, a Scottish trail-builder, drilled six-inch deep holes into the smooth eastern side of the peak. After pounding in iron pegs and fastening ropes to them, he managed to reach the summit. Today, thousands of hikers climb Half Dome by the same route where the National Park Service has now installed a unique cable ladder.

Soon I arrived at Falls Bridge, and just beyond, the junction of the Mist and John Muir trails. It had been recommended that I ascend Mist Trail, and use John Muir Trail for the descent. But this was not possible, as I planned to meet Mary Fran and Jenny coming up the Mist Trail at the end of the day. So, wanting to see both options, I headed up the John Muir Trail. That was a mistake. After a few minutes, I came upon a trail crew-and-pack train. The horses were simply standing on the trail, and the wrangler warned me not to pass. So there I stood. Soon the train began to move, and I trudged along behind 12 horses, not a position I relish. After a while the wrangler stopped again to rest the horses, and there I stood again, unable to pass. It was maddening! This frustrating stop-and-go travel continued all the way to the top of Nevada Falls. At the top of the falls, I rested only briefly before forging up the trail in advance of the horses. It was 9:30 a.m., and I was at last making good time.

After climbing over a rocky crest, I strolled along the Merced River in Little Yosemite Valley. The trail here was flat but sandy, like walking on a beach, and it was a little tiring. I was glad to finally turn uphill toward my objective. The trail climbed gently and surely until I reached a crest and could look down into Tenaya Canyon.

At last I broke out onto a high rocky ridge and Half Dome rose before me in two huge humps. The trail climbed over the first hump in a ragged path constructed roughly of large rocks, and finally the infamous cable ladder came into view.

What a sight it was! From this distance the ladder appeared as a tiny line on the enormous granite dome,

The ladder to the top of Half Dome

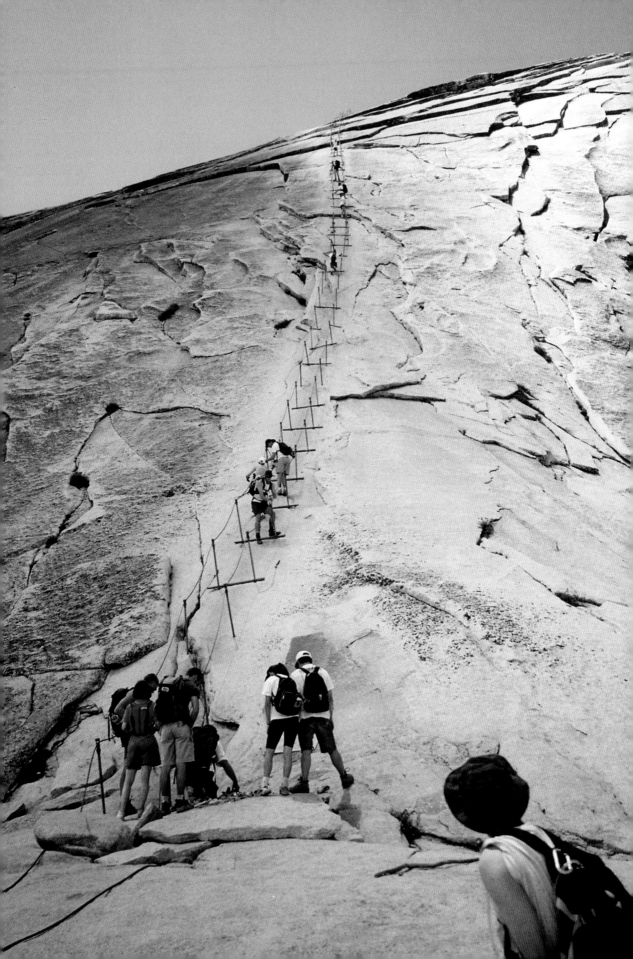

and the line was covered with ants. At the bottom of the ladder was a large crowd of people, many of whom had decided that this was far enough. I made my way directly to the bottom of the ladder and took a short break at 11:30 a.m.

At the bottom of the ladder was a large cache of gloves of all types, colors, and sizes for use on the ladder. Finding two gloves that matched was impossible, so I just settled for two that fit. The look straight up the ladder was intimidating, but this was what I had come for, so I assumed the identity of an ant and took my place in the cue on the ladder. I soon found that my gloves were slipping on the steel cable and were more trouble than they were worth, so I stuck them in my back pocket. Eventually I developed a rhythm: pull hard up the cable to reach the next step, rest five to ten seconds, and then pull again. The ladder was jammed with people, making it necessary to pass others going up, coming down, and just going nowhere. Finally I walked, panting, onto the summit of the Half Dome at 12:30 p.m. The climb from Happy Isles had taken me nearly five hours.

There was a great comradery among those who had achieved the summit, and what a view I was privileged to share with them. The valley was spread out at my feet like a grand cathedral whose roof had been stripped away. The thin plume of Yosemite Falls swayed silently in the wind across the valley. The view straight down the sheer northwest face was stomach-dropping. Royal Robbins, Jerry Gallwas, and Mike Sherrick first climbed this face in 1957, which is still considered one of the great classic climbs of North America. But from this vantage point it looked like madness. To the east I could see Clouds Rest, the Cathedral Range, and the great ramparts of the Sierra Nevada. I gave my camera to someone for a picture, and walked out on the Visor, the great brow that protrudes above the northwest face. All logic told me that it would not choose this point in time to crumble, and yet it was a very unsettling place to stand.

I wanted to stay and see the sunset from this magical place, but the world was calling me back. And so, after lunch, I started back down the cables. Here the gloves proved their real value in the slide down, as they prevented friction burn from the cables.

As I descended the Mist Trail on my return to the valley, I got a better appreciation of the impressive chasm below Little Yosemite Valley. Sweeping around the southern shoulder of Half Dome, the Merced

River has carved a dramatic canyon while plunging over two great waterfalls: Nevada Falls and Vernal Falls. Vernal Falls drops over a ledge in a thundering 317-foot free fall to the rocks below. Nevada Falls is more fluid, meeting a granite face that sweeps it gracefully and smoothly toward its base 597 feet below. Although very different, their beauty and setting make these waterfalls two of the loveliest in America.

I met Mary Fran and Jenny at the top of Vernal Falls at 4 p.m. as planned, and we strolled together back to the Happy Isles Bridge and shuttle bus stop 16 at 5 p.m. The entire hike had taken me nine hours and 15 minutes from start to finish. I was tired, of course, but pleasantly so, not completely exhausted as I had expected. The hike to the summit of Half Dome had met my every expectation. It is a hike unlike any other hike I know, and I could think of none better.

Once on the shuttle bus, I glanced back at this ageless icon of Yosemite Valley, now rising thousands of feet above us. "At the head of the valley, now clearly revealed, stands the Half Dome, the loftiest, most sublime and the most beautiful of all the rocks that guard this glorious temple . . . finely sculptured and poised in calm, deliberate majesty." Thus did John Muir describe Half Dome after first seeing Yosemite Valley, and so it remains today.

DIRECTIONS TO THE TRAIL-HEAD AND TRAIL ROUTE

The trail to Half Dome begins at the Happy Isles Bridge near shuttle bus stop 16. Hikers must use the Yosemite Valley Shuttle Bus, as it is no longer permitted to drive and park at the trailhead. This makes getting a very early start problematic. From Happy Isles Bridge, hike up the left bank of the Merced River 0.8 miles to Falls Bridge for the first view of Vernal

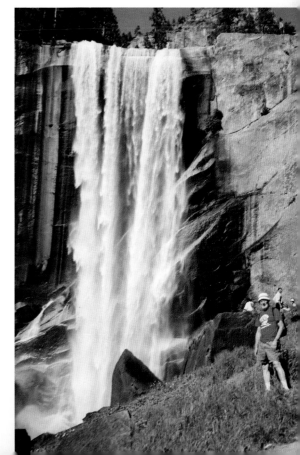

Jack in front of Vernal Falls

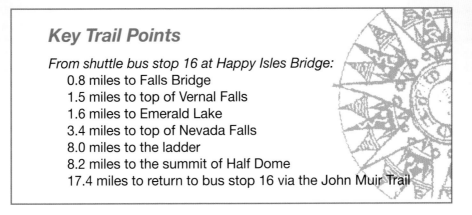

Key Trail Points

From shuttle bus stop 16 at Happy Isles Bridge:
- 0.8 miles to Falls Bridge
- 1.5 miles to top of Vernal Falls
- 1.6 miles to Emerald Lake
- 3.4 miles to top of Nevada Falls
- 8.0 miles to the ladder
- 8.2 miles to the summit of Half Dome
- 17.4 miles to return to bus stop 16 via the John Muir Trail

Falls. Just beyond Falls Bridge hikers must make a choice, since two trails lead to the top of Nevada Falls. Mist Trail is short and steep, affording wonderful close-up views of both falls. It is very possible, depending on wind conditions, to get wet from the spray on this trail. The other choice is John Muir Trail, which switchbacks high up the right slope, and then contours back down to the top of Nevada Falls. John Muir Trail is much gentler, being the one used by pack animals, but is over a mile longer. Either trail may be used. Having hiked both trails, I recommend ascending Mist Trail, which is the more dramatic of the two, and descending the less precarious John Muir Trail at the end of the day when your muscles are spent. The hike using this option is 17.4 miles round-trip. Using the Mist Trail both ways reduces the distance to just over 16.4 miles. In either case, climb to the top of Nevada Falls, 1,870 vertical feet above the trailhead.

From Nevada Falls the trail leads over a rise, then down to the floor of Little Yosemite Valley. Just 1.1 miles beyond Nevada Falls, bear left up the John Muir Trail toward Half Dome. After another 1.5 miles, turn left again on Half Dome Trail. The trail gains the crest of the ridge, and then begins ascending the first hump of the dome itself. The trail here is steep and much more severe. After cresting the first hump, the trail leads over exposed rock to the base of the cable ladder. This will be the stopping point for those with a fear of heights, for the "ladder" rises steeply above, and is not at all as one might imagine it. The ladder consists of two steel cable handrails, with large wooden rungs fastened on the rock about eight feet apart. Even in the best of conditions, the ladder can be frightening. But as the season progresses, rungs get broken and it becomes even more intimidating. Most days the ladder will be jammed with people, some ascending and some descending. Sometimes people just stop, making it necessary to pass, or even climb outside the ladder. Gloves are recommended to prevent friction burn on the cables, especially during the descent. All things considered, the cable ladder to the top of Half Dome should not be underestimated.

Once on the summit, the view of Yosemite Valley is unparalleled. Looking east, the peaks of the Sierra Nevada sweep the horizon in a grand and glorious vista. Plan to spend time on the summit, and muster some courage to stand on the dramatic Visor above the northwest face for a classic picture. To be on the summit of Half Dome is a once-in-a-lifetime experience! Retrace your steps to the trailhead at the Happy Isles Bridge, using either the Mist Trail or the John Muir Trail for the descent.

It would be wise to check the condition of the trail and cable ladder, especially if attempting the hike either very early or late in the season.

Half Dome is especially dangerous when lightning threatens. In July 1985 five hikers made a fateful decision to climb the ladder even as skies darkened and thunder rolled. Once on top, they took shelter in a small cave atop the Visor (see photo on page 50). But a rock cave is no protection in a thunder storm. A powerful lightning bolt struck Half Dome and surged through the cave, killing two and gravely wounding two others. Survivors were saved only by a desperate post-midnight helicopter rescue.

NOTE: For descriptions of weather and wildlife, lodging and camping, and fees and contacts for Yosemite Valley, see those sections for Yosemite Falls Trail on page 49.

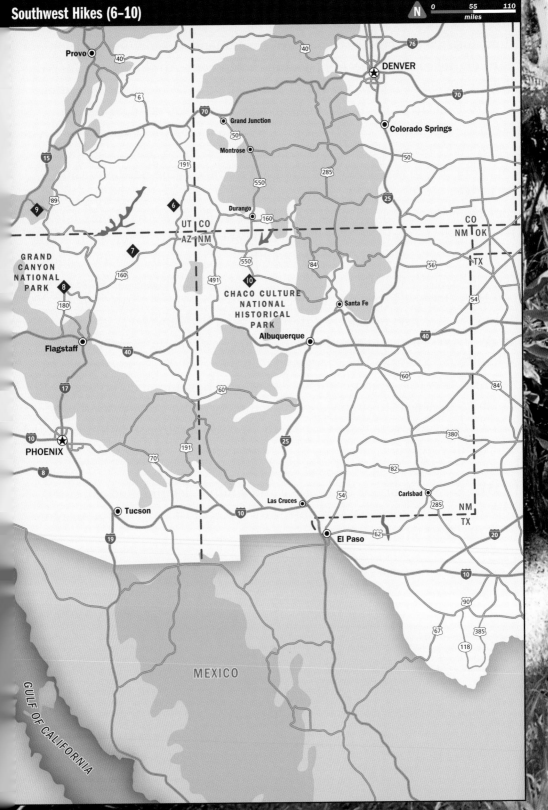

N 0 55 110
miles

Provo · 40

40 · 76

DENVER ★

6

70

Grand Junction · 70

50

Colorado Springs ·

15

Montrose ·

50

550

285

89

9

6

191

Durango · 160

UT CO
AZ NM

25

CO
NM OK

7

550

84

56

TX

GRAND
CANYON
NATIONAL
PARK

160

491

CHACO CULTURE
NATIONAL
HISTORICAL
PARK

Santa Fe ·

54

8

180

Albuquerque ·

Flagstaff · 40

40

60

84

17

60

380

10

191

25

82

PHOENIX ★

70

Las Cruces ·

54

Carlsbad ·

285

NM

8

10

TX

Tucson ·

El Paso · 62

20

19

90

MEXICO

67

385

118

GULF OF CALIFORNIA

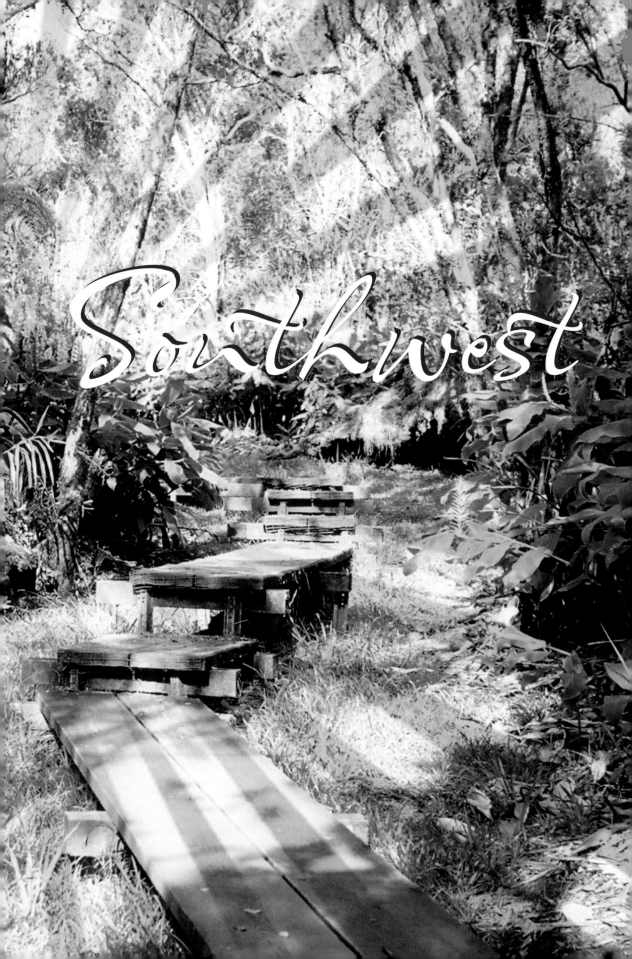

Southwest

06 DEVILS GARDEN LOOP

Location: *Arches National Park, UT*
Distance: *6.7 miles*
Elevation Extremes: *5,025 to 5,530 feet*
Total Elevation Gain: *595 feet*
Difficulty: *Moderate*
Maps: *Mollie Hogans 7.5-minute*
Trailhead Coordinates: *N 38° 46' 59.4" W 109° 35' 42.6"*
UTM 12S 0622000 4293650 [WGS84]

"DESERT SOLITAIRE"

The high desert of southeastern Utah is no place to get careless. I learned that in a bitter lesson 25 years ago when I first hiked Devils Garden Loop with my family. We took too little water, ran out barely halfway around Primitive Loop, and were parched by the time we reached the drinking fountain at the trailhead. I would not make the same mistake again, but others were about to learn the same harsh lesson.

The sun glared down from a cloudless sky that July morning, and it was already sizzling hot in Arches National Park. My family and I loaded up with water and started down the trail at 9:10 a.m. The scene before us was like no other in the world. Rising boldly from the Colorado Plateau in southeastern Utah is a strange and fantastic collection of rock buttes, spires, fins, and arches. Arches National Park contains the greatest density of natural stone arches on the planet—more than 2,000 arches in an area of 119 square miles. Edward Abbey, in his classic book *Desert Solitaire,* described an arch as "A weird, lovely, fantastic object of nature . . . . its significance lies in the power of the odd and unexpected to startle the senses and surprise the mind out of their ruts of habit, to compel us into a reawakened awareness of the wonderful . . . . for a little while we are again able to see, as a child sees, a world of marvels."

Only 20 minutes down the trail we arrived at Landscape Arch. I was pleased to see this spectacular structure still standing. Despite its 306-foot span, it is only about 11 feet thick at its center. It was 5 feet thicker until September 1991 when a 60-foot-long and 4-foot-thick slab crashed down from the underside of the arch's thinnest section. Like living things, arches have a natural life cycle, and it seems likely that Landscape Arch's years are numbered.

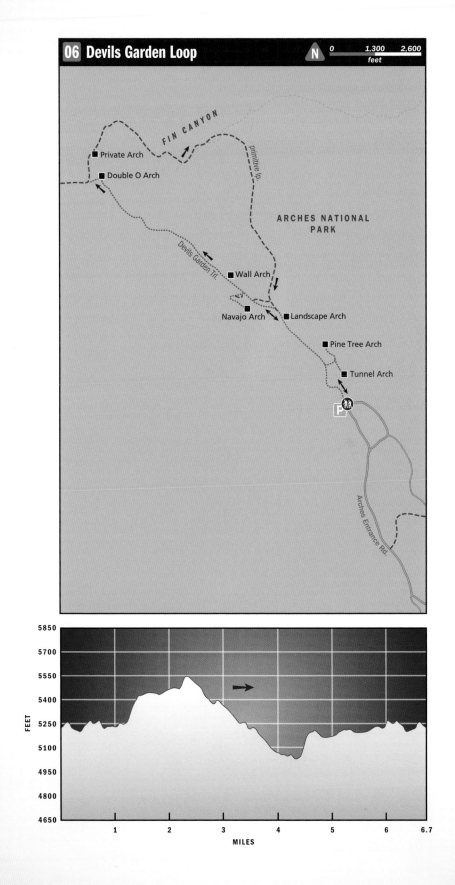

As Mary Fran and Jenny headed back to the comfort of air-conditioning, I continued on the trail toward Double O Arch. After climbing a rugged passageway beneath Wall Arch (*Note:* Wall Arch suddenly collapsed in the summer of 2008), I reached a trail junction and turned left up a side trail. I was rewarded with lovely views of Navajo Arch, a secluded opening hidden between rock fins, and Partition Arch, which offers a stunning view of desert and distant mountains through its opening.

The main trail continued across a high rock fin. A fin is a narrow free-standing slab of rock that is the first step in the development of an arch. Erosion of fins continue over time as water seeps into superficial cracks, widened in turn by freezing and thawing and the action of the wind, until many fins collapse. Others, with just the right combination of hardness and balance, survive and become famous arches. Thus the landscape of arches remains a work in progress.

306-foot-long Landscape Arch

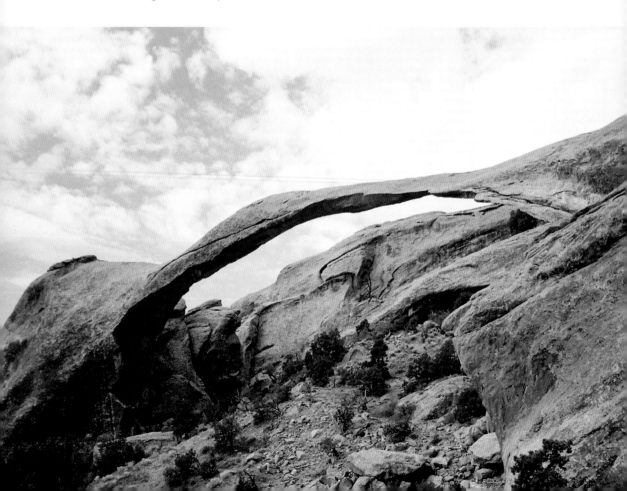

I arrived at Double O Arch at 10:40 a.m. The view of Double O was somewhat spoiled by several hikers who had climbed up into the arch for a rowdy picnic, but the scene was still remarkable with the black tower known as the Dark Angel brooding on the horizon. I indulged in a snack myself before continuing on Primitive Loop.

Here a trail sign warned "Caution, Primitive Trail, Difficult Hiking." Most hikers return here by way of the main trail, but the rewards of Primitive Loop make the effort more than worthwhile. This time I carried two quarts of water plus two cans of soda, enough for this hike despite the blistering midday heat. Primitive Loop continues through dramatic desert landscape and down secret fin canyons, marked only by an occasional rock cairn.

After taking another side trail to secluded Private Arch, I resumed my way along Primitive Loop through Fin Canyon. I was soon startled to be passed by two boys running down the trail clad only in shorts and T-shirts. An older woman followed a few minutes later, apparently trying to keep up and carrying no water. This was no place to be hasty, as following Primitive Loop requires careful vigilance. After about 20 minutes, I noticed the same woman who had passed me wandering about 100 yards off-trail in the desert. After I hailed her, she casually returned to the trail, said a few words in French, and ran off up the trail. I could only shake my head. She could easily have been in serious trouble.

I arrived back at Landscape Arch at noon, and after a final side trip to see Pine Tree Arch and Tunnel Arch, arrived back at the trailhead at 12:30 p.m. It was a memorable trip through a strange and magnificent landscape. For me, as for Edward Abbey, the arches of Arches National Park will always reawaken an "awareness of the wonderful . . . a world of marvels!"

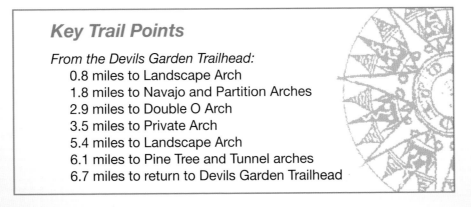

Key Trail Points

From the Devils Garden Trailhead:
- 0.8 miles to Landscape Arch
- 1.8 miles to Navajo and Partition Arches
- 2.9 miles to Double O Arch
- 3.5 miles to Private Arch
- 5.4 miles to Landscape Arch
- 6.1 miles to Pine Tree and Tunnel arches
- 6.7 miles to return to Devils Garden Trailhead

DIRECTIONS TO TRAILHEAD AND TRAIL ROUTE

To reach Devils Garden Trailhead, enter the park at its main entrance on US 191 about 4 miles northwest of Moab, Utah, and follow the park road north 17.7 miles. Water is available at the trailhead, so be sure to take plenty, as well as protection from the glaring sun.

The first 0.8 miles of the trail, which is graveled and well-graded, winds among tall fins to a spectacular view of Landscape Arch. It is one of the longest natural arches in the world, and possibly one of the most fragile. The trail beyond Landscape Arch becomes rougher and more challenging. The trail is sometimes sandy, and sometimes goes across or on top of sandstone fins with sharp drop-offs on either side. Desert sandstone is called slickrock, and can be slippery even when dry.

Only 0.6 miles beyond Landscape Arch, a worthwhile side trail to the left leads to Navajo Arch and Partition Arch. After returning to the main trail, continue on across fins to Double O Arch, a unique combination of one arch above another.

Primitive Loop return trail is significantly more difficult to follow and travel. Primitive Loop can be especially challenging in cold weather when snow or ice can make sections of the trail slick or even impassable. It winds through desert and fin canyons 2.2 miles back to Landscape Arch.

After regaining the main trail at Landscape Arch, take time to visit Pine Tree Arch and Tunnel Arch before returning to Devils Garden Trailhead.

WEATHER AND WILDLIFE

Temperatures in Arches National Park commonly exceed 100°F from June through September. In winters, temperatures often drop below freezing. Temperatures may range 50°F or more in a 24-hour period. Over the course of a year, temperatures at ground level can vary a remarkable 170 degrees. On average, less than ten inches of precipitation dampen the vegetation each year. These environmental extremes have created a unique landscape—stark and unforgiving, with a savage grandeur almost beyond description.

Most mammals in the park are nocturnal. These include desert rodents, skunks, ringtails, foxes, bobcats, and mountain lions. Animals

Lunch at Double O Arch

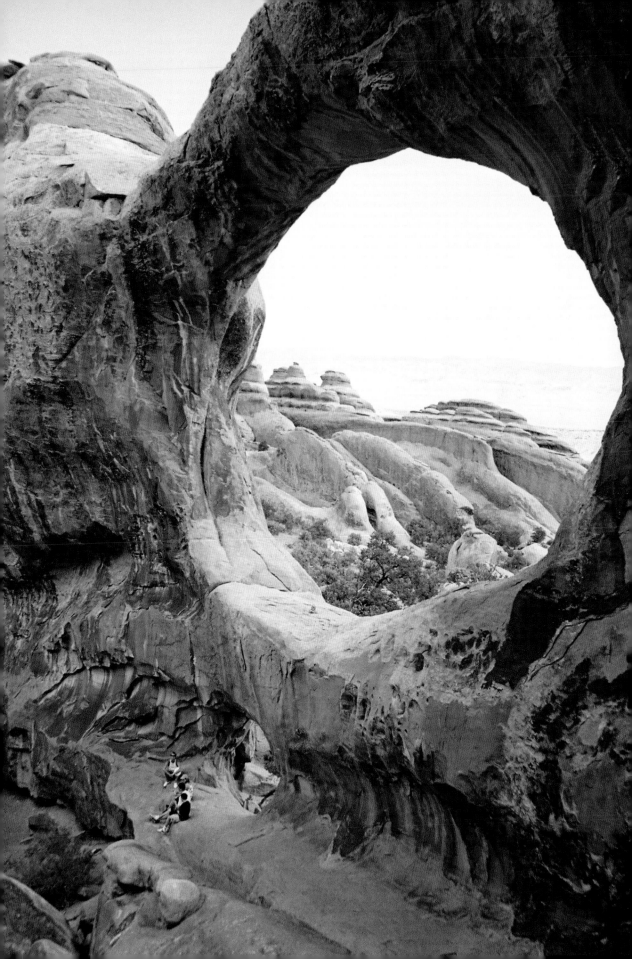

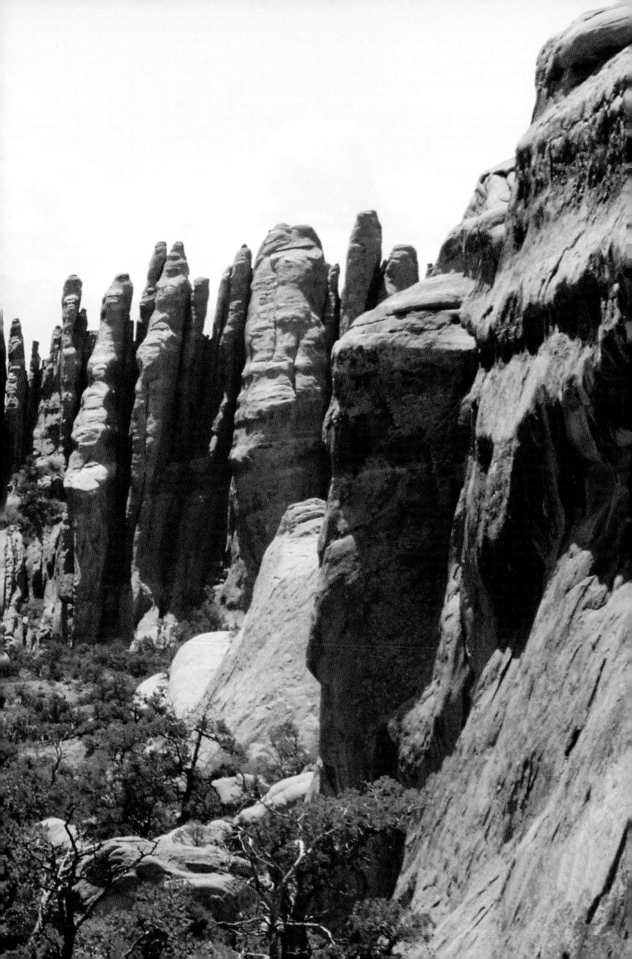

commonly active at dusk include mule deer, coyotes, desert cottontails, and jackrabbits. Animals active during the day in summer are mostly limited to squirrels and lizards. Pets are not permitted on or off trails, and pets left unattended in vehicles during the day can quickly die from heat exhaustion.

There is more vegetation in the park than might be expected considering the heat and lack of precipitation. The dominant plant community here is a pygmy forest: a woodland of pinion and juniper trees. The trees' roots penetrate deep into cracks and fissures in the rock to reach the meager supply of water. Mountain mahogany and cliffrose often grow alongside the trees, taking advantage of their shade and the water funneled off slickrock. Utah juniper, blackbrush, Mormon tea, and yucca plants flourish in the drier habitats of the park.

CAMPING

Sites at the Devils Garden Campground are available for $20 per night and may be reserved online at **www.recreation.gov** or by calling (877) 444-6777. There is an additional booking fee for reservations.

FEES AND CONTACTS

Arches National Park is open 24 hours a day. A fee of $10 per vehicle is charged for a seven-day pass. For more information, write Arches National Park, PO Box 907, Moab, UT 84532-0907, or phone (435) 719-2299. The park Web site is **www.nps.gov/arch**. To get ready for this hike, read the classic book *Desert Solitaire,* written by Edward Abbey when he was a summer ranger at Arches National Park.

Rock Fin Canyon on the
Primitive Trail

07 KEET SEEL

Location: *Navajo National Monument, AZ*
Distance: *16.5 or 17 miles*
Elevation Extremes: *6,325 to 7,270 feet*
Total Elevation Gain: *1,460 feet*
Difficulty: *Very Strenuous*
Maps: *Betatakin Ruin 7.5-minute, Marsh Pass 7.5-minute,
    Keet Seel Ruin 7.5-minute*
Trailhead Coordinates: *N 36° 41' 8.5" W 110° 32' 24.4"
        UTM 12S 0541091 4060099 [WGS84]*

IN THE FOOTSTEPS OF THE ANASAZI

"Be sure to follow the white posts, watch out for quicksand, and take plenty of sunscreen and insect repellant."

The words droned out in a dull monotone from the Navajo woman, who sounded like she had delivered this Keet Seel hike orientation a hundred times before. No matter that Keet Seel is the most perfectly preserved Anasazi ruins in Arizona. For the moment, on this July morning, what caught my attention was the middle thing: Just how does one watch out for quicksand?

But, anxious to get out on the trail, I didn't ask the question. As events would play out, I should have. The morning ranger-guided tour group to Betatakin was about to leave, and I was planning to hitch a ride as far as the Betatakin Ruin parking area, thus saving myself a half mile of walking.

Once at the parking area, I strode off down the trail at 8:40 a.m. ahead of the ranger walk. I felt a sense of excitement and discovery as I descended alone into the mysterious canyons of the Tsegi. I turned left away from the trail to Betatakin at 9:15 a.m., and soon the trail disappeared, the route being marked only by occasional white posts. I crossed Laguna Creek, and then followed the white posts upstream into the obscure Keet Seel Canyon, which splits Skeleton Mesa. At first I tried to keep my feet dry, but it was an impossible task with all the stream crossings, and eventually I just waded across. I passed two lovely waterfalls, the second one about 35 feet high, and arrived at the picnic table below Keet Seel at 12:20 p.m. I could see the ranger guiding four visitors high up in the alcove above, and so I ate lunch while I waited my turn and pondered the mystery of the Anasazi.

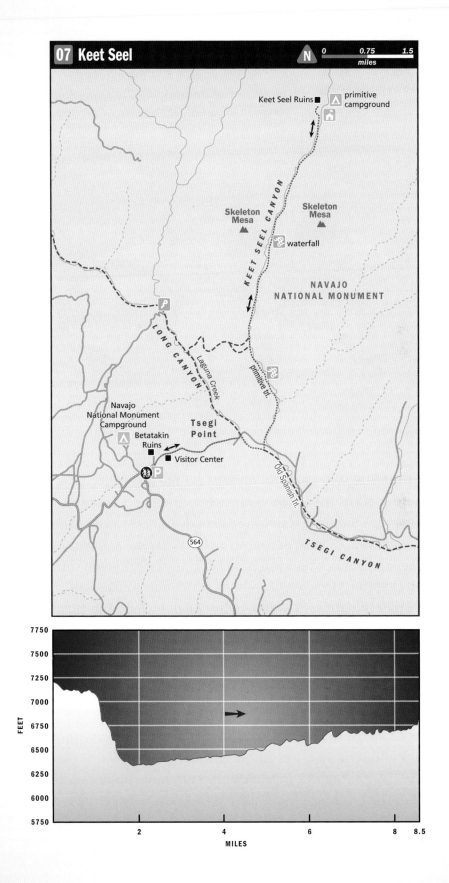

07 Keet Seel

N | 0 | 0.75 | 1.5
miles

Keet Seel Ruins ■ | primitive campground

KEET SEEL CANYON

Skeleton Mesa ▲

Skeleton Mesa ▲

waterfall

NAVAJO NATIONAL MONUMENT

LONG CANYON

Laguna Creek

primitive trl.

Navajo National Monument Campground

Betatakin Ruins ■

Tsegi Point

■ Visitor Center

P

Old Spanish Trl.

564

TSEGI CANYON

FEET

7750
7500
7250
7000
6750
6500
6250
6000
5750

2   4   6   8 8.5
MILES

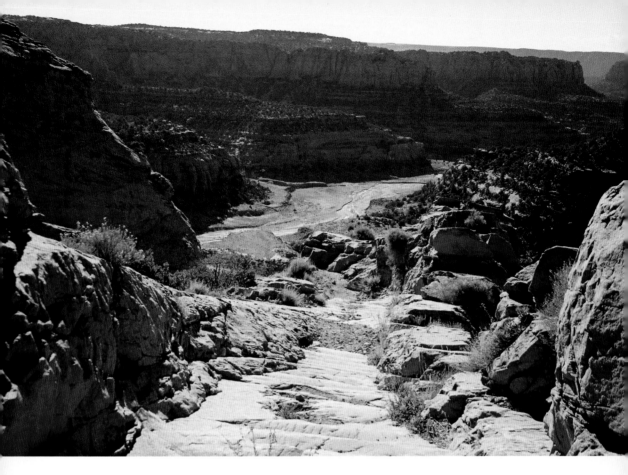

Descending into the canyons of the Tsegi

More than 700 years ago, an ancient people flourished in the Four Corners region of the American Southwest, making a living on this difficult land and building elaborate stone dwellings in the sheltered alcoves of the canyons. These people were the Anasazi, a Navajo word that means "ancient people who were not us." Their best-known communities were located at Mesa Verde, a high plateau in southwestern Colorado. But other magnificent cliff dwellings can be found in the deep and mysterious sandstone canyons of Navajo National Monument in northeastern Arizona. One of these is Keet Seel (meaning "broken pottery"), the second largest cliff dwelling in the world and the best preserved in Arizona. Even from this vantage point the ruin looked spectacular.

After lunch I climbed the 70-foot ladder for my private tour of Keet Seel. Once in the ancient city, I was awestruck by the condition of the dwellings. I had been to other cliff dwellings at Mesa Verde and other locations in the Southwest, but nothing could have prepared me for this. Most of the buildings had their original roofs intact. Some of the walls were of jacal construction: rows of sticks set upright, bound with twigs or string, and covered with plaster. This is typically not a long-lasting type of construction, but here it was, over 700 years old, still standing. The street beneath my feet was littered with corncobs, broken pottery, and pieces of rope. I picked up a piece of rope made from yucca fiber over seven centuries ago and tugged at it—still strong. The ranger picked up a piece of turquoise from the dust. The ghosts of the Anasazi seemed to gaze at us from the dark interiors of the rooms and kivas.

I heard the first peal of thunder just as I completed my tour of the city. "Skeleton Mesa is all slickrock," warned the ranger. "If it rains, the streams could rise five to six feet in a flash. If that happens just climb high up the bank. It'll go back down in three or four hours." I didn't like the sound of that, so I set a fast pace back down Keet Seel Canyon.

I soon had my first encounter with quicksand. It was not as I had imagined. Quicksand forms along the river downstream of large boulders, or where water is welling up from springs. Sometimes, if you're fortunate, you can walk right across it. I was not so lucky. My left foot suddenly began to sink. When I tried to pull it out, my right foot also became trapped. Startled, I fell flat and crawled to the stream bank. I was soon standing safe on the bank, but a little shaken. Unfortunately, my left shoe was still stuck in the sand. After a little hand wringing, I was able to lay a dead Juniper branch down, crawl out on it, and retrieve my shoe from the muck. I continued down the canyon a little wiser, and with a lot more caution!

Soon the sky turned black and the thunder echoed through the canyon walls. I picked up my pace, and crossed Laguna Creek for the last time just as the first raindrops began to fall. I climbed another 200 feet above the creek, and then witnessed an amazing sight. Waterfalls poured off the slickrock into the canyon from every side. A wave of white, foaming water rushed down Long Canyon at breakneck speed, followed by an angry tide of thick red water carrying sticks and other debris. I was truly thankful that I had completed my last stream crossing!

After the thunderstorm, I climbed the trail to Tsegi Point and walked the remaining distance to the Keet Seel parking area, arriving at 5:30 p.m. It had been an amazing day, filled with mysteries of the Anasazi and the natural wonders of the sandstone canyons of Navajo National Monument. I had experienced glorious ancient ruins that few people visit, quicksand, and an exciting flashflood all in one day. This was one of the best hikes of my life.

Key Trail Points

From the trailhead at the Keet Seel parking area:
0.5 miles to Betatakin parking area
2.3 miles to Laguna Creek
3.0 miles to Keet Seel Canyon
6.0 miles to 35-foot waterfall
8.5 miles to Keet Seel
17 miles to return to Keet Seel Parking Area

DIRECTIONS TO TRAILHEAD AND TRAIL ROUTE

Keet Seel can be visited only by a demanding 17-mile hike through deep and secretive canyons. The route is marked only by mileage posts every 0.5 miles, and is made difficult by numerous stream crossings, stifling midday temperatures, violent summer thunderstorms, and quicksand. Keet Seel is open daily from Memorial Day weekend to Labor Day weekend. Site tours normally start around 9:30 a.m., and are conducted throughout the day as people arrive. Keet Seel cannot be visited without a permit, and reservations are limited to 20 persons per day. Reservations may be made no more than five months in advance

Keet Seel ruin

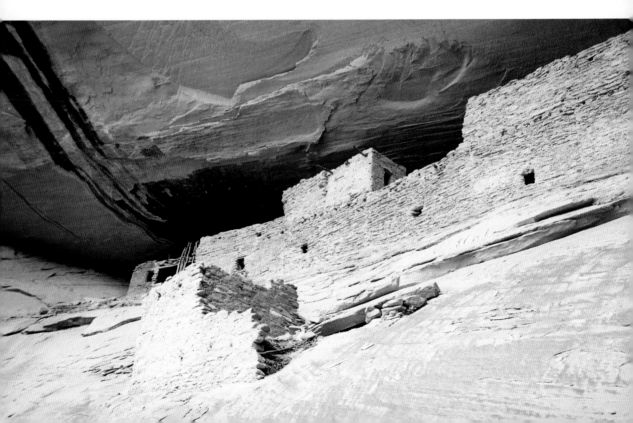

of the hike, and must be reconfirmed no later than one week before the visit or the permit will be cancelled. Reservations must be made in person or by telephone at (928) 692-2700. A few openings may be available six days before a visit on a first-come, first-serve basis from unconfirmed reservations, or the day of the hike from those who fail to arrive by 9 a.m. Hiking to Keet Seel without a permit, or off-trail hiking in the surrounding canyons is strictly prohibited by law. Every hiker to Keet Seel must attend an orientation program, either at 4 p.m. the day before the hike or at 8:15 the morning of the hike.

Hikers often start the long hike to Keet Seel at sunrise, but strong hikers can also complete the hike after the morning orientation program. To reach the trailhead, first exit the Navajo National Monument Visitor Center parking lot and turn right to the Keet Seel parking area near the overflow campground. From here Keet Seel is 8.5 miles away (17 miles round-trip). The hike can be shortened a little by driving through a gate to the Betatakin parking area 0.5 miles ahead, but this can be done only if accompanied by a park ranger.

From the Keet Seel parking area, hike past the Betatakin parking area and toilet. From here mileage posts every 0.5 miles mark the remaining distance to Keet Seel. At the 7-mile mark, the trail descends about 1,000 feet from Tsegi Point into the wild and remote canyons of Tsegi (Navajo for "Rock Canyon"). At the bottom of the first set of switchbacks, the trail branches to Betatakin and Keet Seel. Follow the path to the left toward Laguna Creek below. A large white post will be found just before reaching the creek. Stand at this post and look downstream and you will see the next white post, which will guide you out of the main canyon and into a tributary canyon. Continue following posts in this fashion into Keet Seel Canyon. It will be necessary to cross streams several times, so plan to get your feet wet. You will encounter two waterfalls at mileposts 2.5 and 5.5. These can be passed by short side trails on the right, but do not take any other trails out of the canyon or into surrounding canyons. Pass the Keet Seel Primitive Campground just beyond a grove of elders at milepost 0.5, and continue up the left bank to the monument boundary fence. Here you will find a picnic table in an oak grove and the first spectacular view of Keet Seel.

Upon arrival, contact the resident park ranger and arrange for a tour. No one may enter the ruins without the ranger, and no more than five people may tour Keet Seel at any one time. Day hikers have priority for tours in order to return within the day. Sport sandals or tennis shoes with nonaggressive treads are required to lessen the impact on the fragile ruins.

Once in Keet Seel, the scale and state of preservation of the ruin are stunning. Several tons of fill lie behind a great retaining wall to create a street running the length of the alcove—an impressive engineering feat. Streets are unusual in Anasazi cliff dwellings, and Keet Seel has three. The city also has four different types of kivas, probably an indication of a diverse population. Several granaries were filled with corn before they left, as though they expected to return.

By the year 1290 AD, Keet Seel housed about 125 to 150 people. More than 150 rooms stretched beneath the long overhang, and several more rested on the ground below. Then, with no apparent explanation, all the inhabitants left everything they couldn't carry—homes, crops, and belongings—and mysteriously moved on. Today Keet Seel remains a superb testament to Anasazi skill and culture. Its remarkable preservation

35-foot waterfall in Keet Seel Canyon

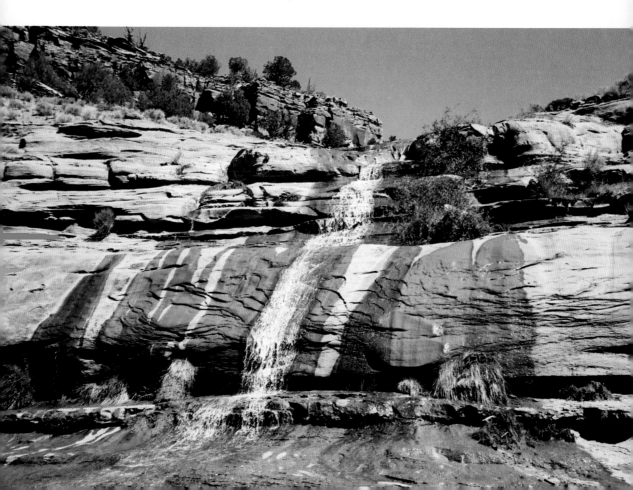

is due to its relatively inaccessible location in the Tsegi Canyon system of Navajo National Monument. The Navajo intentionally avoid the cliff dwellings lest they provoke the ghosts of ancient people who lived there.

After touring these magnificent ruins, return to the Keet Seel parking area by the same route in reverse. Respect these ruins and this beautiful land by taking nothing with you and leaving no mark behind.

WEATHER AND WILDLIFE

Summer weather can be hot and changeable. Violent thunderstorms are common from July to September, and flash floods are not unusual. Do not attempt to cross streams during flash floods! Wait on higher ground for the water to subside. Midday temperatures in the canyon can exceed 100°F. To avoid excessive exposure, plan to hike in the early morning, wear a hat, seek shade, and, if necessary, drench your clothing with water. Take plenty of water, since stream water is contaminated from cattle and other animal feces. Water filters do not remove viruses. Watch out for rockfall and collapsing dirt banks along creeks and gullies, and, of course, watch out for quicksand.

Note that during the summer the Navajo Nation, including Navajo National Monument, is on mountain daylight savings time (MDST), and is therefore one hour ahead of all other Arizona locations.

CAMPING

The monument has two campgrounds, Sunset View Campground and Canyon View Campground, with a total of 48 sites available first come, first serve. Camping just below Keet Seel is also available to those who do not wish to complete this hike in a single day. There is no lodging available in Navajo National Monument. Motels and other services can be found in Kayenta, Arizona, about 25 miles east of the monument.

FEES AND CONTACTS

Entrance into the monument and campgrounds is free. The mandatory orientation program is given at the Monument Visitor Center, open from 8 a.m. until 5 p.m., Monday through Friday, and from 8 a.m. until 7 p.m. on weekends. For more information, write Navajo National Monument, HC-71 Box 3, Tonalea, AZ 86044-9704, or phone (928) 672-2700. The park Web site is **www.nps.gov/nava.** The park radio station, AM 1610, broadcasts 24 hours a day with the latest park information.

08 SOUTH KAIBAB–BRIGHT ANGEL LOOP

Location: *Grand Canyon National Park, AZ*
Distance: *14.7–15.5 miles*
Elevation Extremes: *7,260 to 2,450 feet*
Total Elevation Gain: *4,950 feet*
Difficulty: *Very Strenuous*
USGS Maps: *Phantom Ranch 7.5-minute, Grand Canyon 7.5-minute*
Trailhead Coordinates: *N 36° 3' 5.1" W 112° 5' 1.8"*
UTM 12S 0402378 3990196 [WSG84]

INTO THE ABYSS

I stood on the edge of the great abyss, the frail beam of my headlamp disappearing into the inky blackness below. The only hint of civilization was the tiny orange glow of a single light at the North Rim Lodge about 10 miles away across the canyon. A hike from the rim of the Grand Canyon to the river and back is never to be taken lightly, least of all in midsummer when daytime temperatures in the depths of the canyon can be dangerous. I felt excited and more than a little intimidated by the hike before me.

The Grand Canyon! Its very name invokes images of immense scale, timeless beauty, unforgettable adventure, even reverence. This natural marvel is inspiring, intimidating, wonderful and terrible, immense and intimate, magnificent and dreadful, frightening and comforting. As John Wesley Powell, leader of the first expedition party to descend the Colorado River into "the great unknown" said, ". . . it is the most sublime spectacle on earth!"

Today, more than 5 million people visit the Grand Canyon every year, but most only walk to one or more viewpoints and draw a deep breath. Few visitors venture below the rim to understand and experience the canyon on its own terms. Certainly the National Park Service goes to great lengths to discourage tourists from descending far into the canyon, especially in summer, and for good reason. Temperatures on the rims seldom become unbearably hot. The inner gorge, on the other hand, can be torrid, with highs in July averaging 106°F. Visitors hiking down into the canyon often fail to appreciate the effort needed to climb back up thousands of feet to the rim in stifling heat. As a result, about 250 people

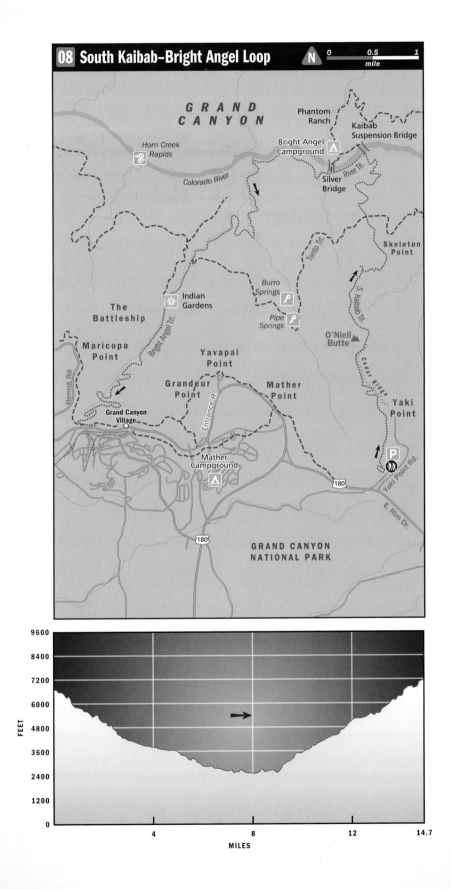

08 South Kaibab–Bright Angel Loop

N — 0 0.5 1 mile

GRAND CANYON

Phantom Ranch

Kaibab Suspension Bridge

Horn Creek Rapids

Bright Angel Campground

Colorado River

Silver Bridge

River Trl.

Tonto Trl.

Skeleton Point

Burro Springs

Indian Gardens

Pipe Springs

The Battleship

S. Kaibab Trl.

O'Niell Butte

Bright Angel Trl.

Maricopa Point

Yavapai Point

Grandeur Point

Mather Point

Cedar Ridge

Yaki Point

Hermit Rd.

Entrance R.

Grand Canyon Village

Mather Campground

Yaki Point Rd.

180

180

E. Rim Dr.

GRAND CANYON NATIONAL PARK

FEET

9600
8400
7200
6000
4800
3600
2400
1200
0

MILES

4   8   12   14.7

need to be evacuated by helicopter from the depths of the canyon each year, and many die from dehydration and heat exhaustion. A rim-to-river-and-back hike ideally should not be attempted in the summer months. Hikers should carry plenty of water and be adequately prepared, both mentally and physically, for the challenge ahead.

I had to avoid the scorching temperatures of midday, so I left my rental car at a small picnic area just past the turnoff to Yaqui Point at 2:30 a.m. I turned on my headlamp and walked past barriers to South Kaibab Trailhead. Regrettably, this strategy would lengthen my hike to 15.5 miles, and I would miss the spectacular views of the canyon from the upper South Kaibab Trail, but I felt I had no choice. If all went well, I would be at the river just after dawn, be out of the inner gorge shortly thereafter, and finish my hike up Bright Angel Trail by 1 p.m.

I descended into the dark abyss at 2:45 a.m. There was no moon, and the stars glistened like a thousand jewels. The rocks and trail in front of me glowed dimly from the light of my headlamp, but always present on one side was the black, ominous void of the canyon. Aside from the sound of my boots on the trail, the silence was overwhelming.

I reached Cedar Ridge in darkness at about 3 a.m., and encountered my first problem. Cedar Ridge is a popular tourist destination, and trails run helter-skelter in every direction. It took me several minutes, but eventually I found the right path and continued down South Kaibab Trail in the dark. At Skeleton Point I heard the first distant but unmistakable roar of rapids. It was 4:20 a.m. A faint orange glow tinted the morning sky, and a new point of light, which I assumed to be at Phantom Ranch, appeared in the inky depths below. I felt very small and alone.

I arrived at the junction with Tonto Trail at 5:15 a.m. and took my first rest. There was a small building here and a phone for emergency use. Despite getting lost for a while at Cedar Ridge, I was pleased with my progress.

I descended below the Tipoff, and turned left onto River Trail at 6:15 a.m. Thankfully it was still cool in the inner gorge. I crossed the Bright Angel Suspension Bridge to the other side, made my way down to the river, and ceremonially dunked my hat in the muddy Colorado. On this same river in 1869, John Wesley Powell, a self-taught biologist and Civil War veteran with one arm, led the first descent of the Grand Canyon by boat. His 26-day epic in the canyon is the stuff of legends

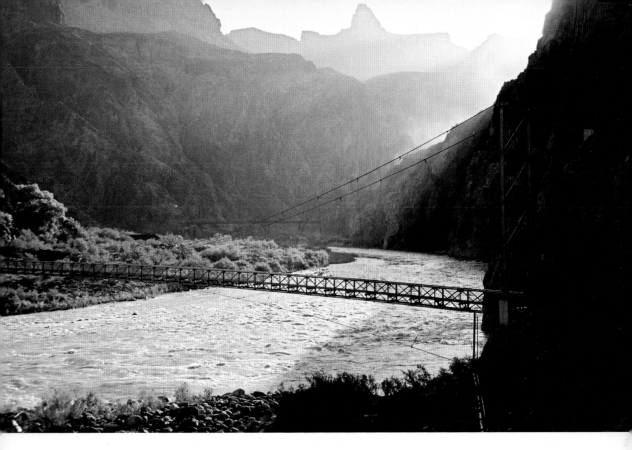

Bright Angel Suspension Bridge across the Colorado River

and remains one of my favorite stories. While I was re-crossing the
suspension bridge, two blue rafts coasted silently beneath me retracing
Powell's historic journey. The passengers waved a giddy hello.

In the steely light of dawn, the grandeur of the canyon was fully
revealed. Ancient towers of stone—Zoroaster Temple, Isis Temple, and
Wotan's Throne—rose thousands of feet above me. Sunlight poured into
the canyon in a drama of light and space. And here, the eternal flow of
the river lent an even more surreal quality to the scene. There are only
a few places where the river can actually be seen from the rim of the
canyon. The river's presence and power can be perceived from the rim
only by its handiwork; this is the same river that, over countless mil-
lennia and grain by grain, carved this magnificent edifice.

The River Trail downriver from the suspension bridge was sandy,
making progress slow and tiring. Moreover, the sun was now glaring
in the sky. The inner gorge was already beginning to heat up. I saw
the two blue rafts tied up below the trail at Pipe Creek Rapids. They
were changing crews. Those who had come this far were hiking up the
Bright Angel Trail, and new passengers were hiking down to raft the
river downstream. I was glad to turn up a shady canyon on the Bright

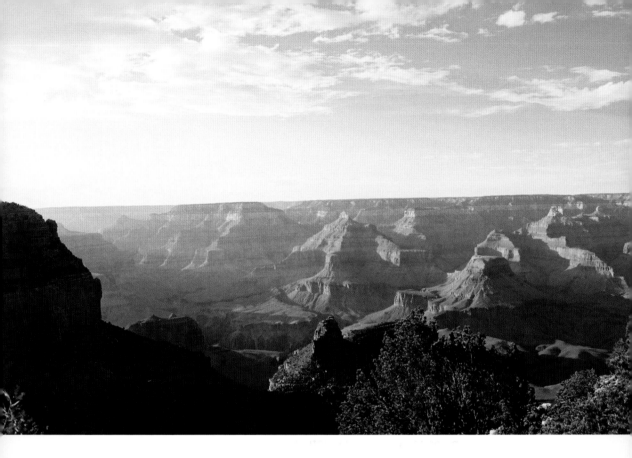

The Grand Canyon from the South Rim

Angel Trail, and took only a brief break at the River Resthouse, a small wooden shelter with another emergency phone.

After a series of steep switchbacks, the trail leveled out and I passed the remains of the Bright Angel Mine, active from the late 1880s to 1908, on my left. The trail then entered a very quiet, enjoyable section of trail—the shady cleft of Indian Garden Creek with its many caves and ledges cut into the Tapeats Sandstone. I arrived at the booming metropolis of Indian Gardens at 9:20 a.m., where the silence I had enjoyed so far was broken. A mule train was tied up nearby, and the benches were full of noisy riders and hikers. Everyone seemed anxious to share their experience, and was amazed to hear that I had come from rim to river and back, since the park rangers told them that this was impossible. I took a long rest at Indian Gardens and filled my water bottles. A thermometer mounted on a tree read a balmy 98°F as I headed up toward the rim. I was lucky. This day was a little cooler than most.

I was on schedule, and so allowed myself a brief rest at the Three-Mile Resthouse, where a thermometer read a comfortable 90°F, and again at the Mile-and-a-Half Resthouse. Above the Mile-and-a-Half

Resthouse, I passed many hikers who had overestimated their abilities and were now struggling in the heat to regain the canyon rim. I met Mary Fran coming down the trail near the top and arrived at the Bright Angel Trailhead just after 1 p.m. I could not have been more content.

No collection of great American hikes would be complete without a hike into the magnificent Grand Canyon of the Colorado River. As the hiker descends into the abyss, the history of the canyon opens up like a book, and glorious temples of rock rise on all sides. It is timeless in its beauty, demanding in its challenge, and absolutely unique in the world. It is the Grand Canyon!

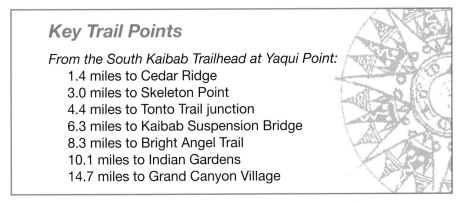

Key Trail Points

From the South Kaibab Trailhead at Yaqui Point:
1.4 miles to Cedar Ridge
3.0 miles to Skeleton Point
4.4 miles to Tonto Trail junction
6.3 miles to Kaibab Suspension Bridge
8.3 miles to Bright Angel Trail
10.1 miles to Indian Gardens
14.7 miles to Grand Canyon Village

DIRECTIONS TO TRAILHEAD AND TRAIL ROUTE

South Kaibab Trail is recommended for a morning descent since it offers no water and little shade. Climbing it in hot weather is foolish. The well-traveled and ultra-manicured Bright Angel Trail is a better choice for the ascent, as it is tucked down into shady canyons and provides several rest and water stops along the way.

The South Kaibab Trailhead is located on the west side of Yaqui Point, about 4 miles east of Grand Canyon Village off Arizona Route 64. Unfortunately, Yaqui Point is closed to automobile traffic, so a car must be left 0.75 miles from the trailhead on AZ 64. From mid-March until mid-October there is a free hiker's shuttle that runs between Bright Angel Lodge and the trailhead at Yaqui Point. The hiker's shuttle could be used for a late start, or can be used to retrieve a car after the hike. From the trailhead, descend a series of steep switchbacks past spectacular Ooh Aah Point to Cedar Ridge, a popular day-hike destination. Leave the tired tourists behind and continue the descent to Skeleton Point and your first view of the mighty Colorado River far below. Descending beneath Skeleton Point, cross the Tonto Trail and reach the Tipoff at the edge of the dark inner gorge. Finally, reach the river at the Kaibab Suspension Bridge 6.3 miles from the trailhead.

Just above the Kaibab Suspension Bridge, turn left on the River Trail, walk past the Bright Angel Suspension Bridge (also known as the Silver Bridge), and join the Bright Angel Trail at Pipe Creek Rapids 2 miles downriver from the South Kaibab Trail. Leaving the river, turn up the Bright Angel Trail and hike past the River Resthouse to Indian Gardens. This section of trail gains about 1,300 feet in 1.8 miles. Indian Gardens is a green oasis where hordes of hikers, down from Grand Canyon Village, rest on benches in the shade of massive cottonwood trees. Drinking water is available here and also at two resthouses on the way up to the rim, located 4.6 miles and 3,100 feet above Indian Gardens.

WEATHER AND WILDLIFE

Fall is usually dry and temperatures moderate in the canyon, making this the season of choice for hiking below the rim. Winter conditions on the South Rim can be extreme, with snow, icy roads and trail conditions, and possible road closures. Spring is typically warm, breezy to windy, and dry with little precipitation.

Common animal sightings include elk, coyotes, ringtails, and skunks. Bobcat, gray fox, and mountain lion sightings are more rare. Mule deer and bighorn sheep have also rebounded since the removal of 500 feral burros in the 1980s. One of the great thrills of the Grand Canyon is to see endangered California condors soaring over the South Rim. Condors are the largest land birds in North America, having a nine-foot wingspan. In 1966, six condors were released at the Vermilion Cliffs north of the canyon, and today there are about 60 birds in Arizona, where they are finally beginning to nest and reproduce.

LODGING AND CAMPING

Some may prefer to split this difficult hike into two days. This can be done with an overnight at either the Bright Angel Campground or Phantom Ranch, located about

Sunrise at the bottom of the Grand Canyon

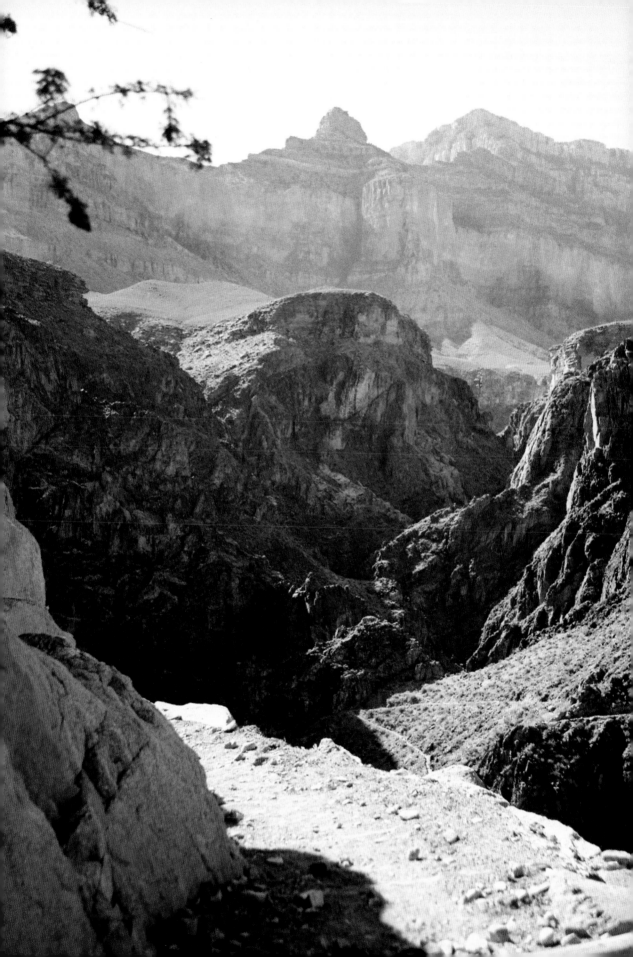

0.5 miles across the river on the North Kaibab Trail. Cabins at Phantom Ranch often sell out on the first day of availability, 11 months ahead. The nine simple cabins, constructed with rocks from Bright Angel Creek, stand peacefully under the shade of cottonwood trees. The cabins were constructed in the 1920s and 1930s, and each contains four to ten bunk beds. Four ten-person dorms, each with its own shower facilities, were constructed for hikers in the early 1980s. Generous meals are served there, and guests are roused at 5 a.m. for an early start to escape the midday heat. Reservations can be made at (303) 297-2757.

There are six lodges within the park on the South Rim, and several other motels are located just outside the park at Tusayan. The Bright Angel Lodge, located at the Bright Angel Trailhead, is a personal favorite of mine. Advance reservations are recommended, especially for the busy summer season. Reservations for any of the park lodges can be made with Xanterra Parks & Resorts at (303) 297-2757, (888) 297-2757, or **www.grandcanyonlodges.com.**

The large Mather Campground is a popular choice on the South Rim. Mather is open year-round with 320 campsites, and a seven-day limit. Mather Campground requires a reservation from March 1 through November 30 and operates on a first-come, first-serve basis the rest of the year. Campsites are $18 per night. Reservations can be made six months in advance at (877) 444-6777 or online at **www.recreation.gov.**

FEES AND CONTACTS

The entrance fee for Grand Canyon National Park is $25 per vehicle for a seven-day pass. Pets must be leashed and are permitted on trails above the rim, but are not allowed below the rim.

For more information, write Grand Canyon National Park, PO Box 129, Grand Canyon, AZ 86023, or phone (928) 638-7888. The park Web site is at **www.nps.goc/grca.**

Done ♡

09 ZION NARROWS

> **Location:** *Zion National Park, UT*
> **Distance:** *15.4 miles*
> **Elevation Extremes:** *4,480 to 5,890 feet*
> **Total Elevation Gain:** *None*
> **Difficulty:** *Very Strenuous*
> **USGS Maps:** *Straight Canyon 7.5-minute, Clear Creek Mountain 7.5-minute, Temple of Sinawava 7.5-minute*
> **Trailhead Coordinates:** *N 37° 23' 12.5" W 112° 50' 18.7"*
> *UTM 12S 0337230 4139360 [WGS84]*

THE DARK UNKNOWN

A series of spectacular stair-stepping plateaus known as the Grand Staircase crowns the high country of southern Utah. Midway into this Grand Staircase, several glorious sandstone temples soar into the clear Utah sky. In 1847, Mormon scouts first entered this remarkable place and named it Zion, a Hebrew word meaning a rocky place of holy sanctuary. Hidden deep within these sandstone temples, the Virgin River drops an amazing 8,000 feet over about 160 miles, one of the steepest river gradients in North America. Here the river has sliced straight down through the sandstone like a knife, forming a dark and foreboding slot canyon up to 2,000 feet deep, and at times only 20 to 30 feet wide. This is recognized as one of the most dramatic and challenging hikes in America. It is called the Zion Narrows.

Most visitors to the park hike only a short distance into the Narrows from the trailhead at the Temple of Sinawava. Many hikers try to reach Orderville Canyon, 1.5 miles upstream, and a few push on to Big Springs at 3.5 miles. Only the most adventurous and hardy attempt the grueling 15.4-mile journey through the entire length of the mysterious Zion Narrows.

I had longed to hike the entire Zion Narrows ever since I walked upstream to Orderville Canyon nearly 20 years ago. I was awestruck! Now I was finally getting my wish. My excitement intensified as the Utah sky gradually changed from deep rose to azure blue. I was riding the Zion Rocky Mountain Guide shuttle from the Zion Canyon Visitor Center to Chamberlain's Ranch. The road deteriorated into deep ruts near the ranch, and I was glad I didn't ask anyone to drive me to the trailhead. Riding with me in the shuttle were four other travelers. A

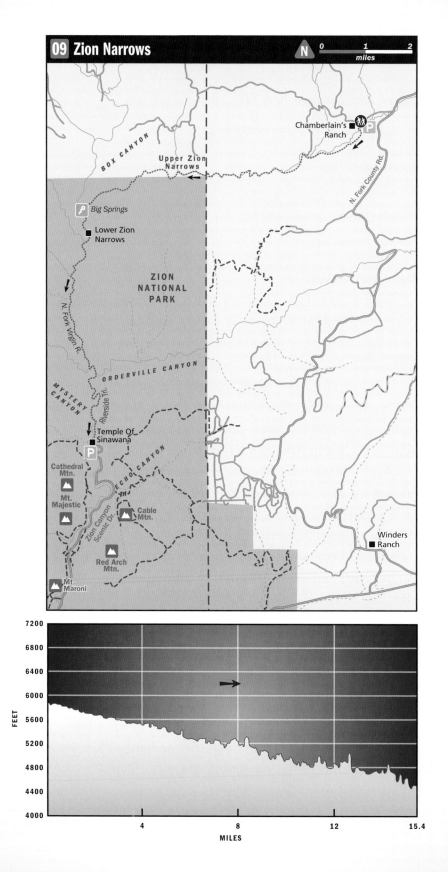

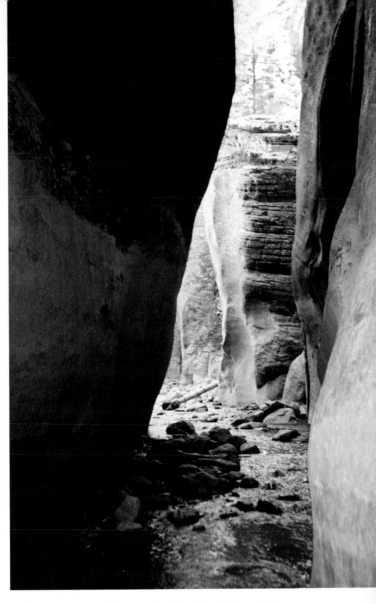

The Upper Zion Narrows

few backpackers were camping in the canyon overnight, but we would be the only day-hikers in the Narrows this day.

The four-wheel-drive Suburban skidded to a stop at the parking lot that marked the trail-head, and we all anx-iously piled out. It was 7 a.m., and the early morn-ing air was clear and crisp. An older man, who was acting as unofficial guide for the other three younger hikers, said "We've GOT to get to the river before nine o'clock!" and off they ran like a pack of rabbits. That pace was much too fast for me, so I thought I'd plod along and wait for the tortoise-and-hare effect to set in.

After about 3 miles walking through easy meadows, the canyon walls began to rise around me as I entered the dark gorge of the Upper Narrows Canyon. At times the canyon was so narrow that I could reach out and touch both walls at once. At first the flow in the river was small, so wading was relatively easy. But after a few miles I found myself look-ing straight down a 15-foot waterfall. I was perplexed. Where was the route downstream? Then I noticed a narrow cleft through the sandstone to my left. Sure enough, the cleft led through a passage in the rock to a gradual descent down a sandy bank and into a pool below the waterfall.

After another mile downstream I passed a boundary sign into Zion National Park. Here the canyon began to widen out, and I noticed the first of 12 established campsites above the Virgin River. I next passed the four "hares," who were slowed down considerably by deep stream crossings and slippery rocks. I paused for lunch and a rest at noon at campsite 4. For a moment I regretted that I was not spending the night in this unique and supremely wild setting.

Just after campsite 12 I passed Big Springs, a lush hanging garden on the right wall, and entered the Lower Zion Narrows. The canyon suddenly took on a grand, yet threatening quality. Both canyon walls rose straight up from the water, and after curiously bowing slightly out, narrowed even more to soar hundreds of feet to the sky above. Sunlight reached the depths of the canyon only on occasion when the angle of the sun perfectly matched the narrow opening through the rock. I could not help imagining what it would be like in a sudden thunderstorm with millions of gallons of water pouring off the slickrock above and coursing down through this defile. Occasionally I could see a log, once part of a malevolent wave of flood debris, wedged tightly between the walls 30 feet above the riverbed. Not a pretty thought.

At one point a deep pool blocked my way. I made my way carefully along a high ledge in an attempt to bypass the pool, as I had done a few

The Three Patriarchs in Zion National Park

times before, but I soon found myself in trouble. I was on a narrow, slippery ledge high above the water and in serious danger of plunging into the very pool I hoped to avoid. I carefully retreated and was happy to wade into the waist-deep but not dangerous water.

Just above Orderville Canyon, I rounded a bend and was surprised to see a dozen people frolicking in the water. From this point on, the hike took on the quality of a raucous carnival. Literally hundreds of people of all ages, shapes, and sizes played in the river.

I took a few minutes to walk up Orderville Canyon, a small branch canyon on the left. This side slot is even narrower, darker, and more extraordinary than the main canyon. Often both walls can be touched at the same time. Sunlight almost never reaches the bottom of this thin slot. Even though I was tired at this point, the side trip was well worth the effort.

After exploring Orderville Canyon a few hundred feet, I walked down to the end of my hike at the Riverside Trail at 4:45 p.m. Mary Fran and Jenny were waiting for me in the river.

The Zion Narrows was one of the best hikes of my life. Walking in the shadow of these soaring walls, sandstone grottos, and hanging gardens was a truly unforgettable wilderness experience. I quietly resolved to search out and hike other magnificent slot canyons of the Southwest. These narrows engendered a feeling of isolation, trepidation, and grandeur that I have felt nowhere else.

Key Trail Points

From the trailhead at Chamberlain's Ranch:
- 4.0 miles to Upper Zion Narrows
- 8.3 miles to Zion National Park boundary
- 10.9 miles to Big Springs and Lower Zion Narrows
- 12.9 miles to Orderville Canyon
- 14.4 miles to Riverside Trail
- 15.4 miles to the Temple of Sinawava shuttle stop

DIRECTIONS TO TRAILHEAD AND TRAIL ROUTE

The trailhead at Chamberlain's Ranch can be accessed by running a car shuttle, or by using a commercial ride service. The trailhead is a one-and-a-half hour drive from the visitor center along paved and dirt roads. The final section of dirt road may be impassable when wet, even for four-wheel-drive vehicles. In good weather, passage over the last mile of road may be difficult for standard front- or rear-wheel-drive passenger cars. To reach the trailhead in your own car, drive 2.5 miles east on Route 9 from the east entrance of the park. Turn left and continue 18 miles to a small wooden bridge that crosses the North Fork of the Virgin River. Turn left after crossing the bridge and continue 0.5 miles to the gate of Chamberlain's Ranch. Pass through the gate (be sure to close the gate behind you) and travel another 0.5 miles to a parking lot marked by a National Park Service trail register. Alternatively, Zion Rocky Mountain Guides, (435) 772-3303, runs a commercial shuttle leaving the visitor center at 6 a.m. to Chamberlain's Ranch for a $20 fee.

From the trailhead, walk downstream following a four-wheel-drive road through pasture for 2.5 miles. The road disappears beyond an old cabin. From this point there is no trail: the route is the river and the riverbed. A walking stick is highly recommended to help maintain balance and lessen the chances of injury and fatigue, but do not cut a tree or bush in the park or on the ranch. Walking sticks can usually be found at an informal depository along the Riverside Walk, or may be purchased or rented in town. Enter the dark Upper Zion Narrows at 4 miles. The canyon becomes broader from about 8 to 10.5 miles where there are 12 numbered campsites, each located above the high-water mark of the river. The shadowy Lower Zion Narrows Canyon is entered after 10.9 miles.

Orderville Canyon, a spectacularly narrow side slot, is passed after another 2 miles, and the paved end of Riverside Trail is reached 1.5 miles beyond that. The final mile brings hikers to the Zion Canyon shuttle stop at the Temple of Sinawava. Be sure to plan your hike so that you do not miss the last shuttle. In summer, the shuttle runs with 15-minute service until 9 p.m., and every 30 minutes between 9 and 11 p.m. The shuttle can be used to return to the Zion Canyon Visitor Center.

Do not underestimate the Zion Narrows hike. There is no maintained trail, and at least 60 percent of the hike is spent wading or sometimes swimming in the river. The current is swift, the water cold, and the rocks underfoot slippery. These conditions make this hike more tiring than one might expect based solely on the distance. Flash flooding and hypothermia are constant dangers. In the 1960s, a sudden flash flood in the canyon caught 26 hikers, drowning five. Good planning, proper equipment, and sound judgment are essential for a safe and successful hike through the Narrows. Make safety your highest priority.

WEATHER AND WILDLIFE

Spring in Zion brings unpredictable weather with stormy, wet days. Precipitation peaks in March. Summer days in the valley are hot with cool nights. Thunderstorms are common from mid-July to mid-September. Fall days are usually clear and mild with chilly nights. Winters in the valley are fairly mild, with snow in the higher elevations. Flash floods can occur at any time, but are more common in midsummer and early fall. From November through May, trips through the Narrows require wetsuits or drysuits and special cold-weather preparation.

Common animals in Zion include coyotes, gray foxes, nocturnal ringtail cats, and skunks. Mule deer and wild turkeys commonly graze

The Lower Zion Narrows

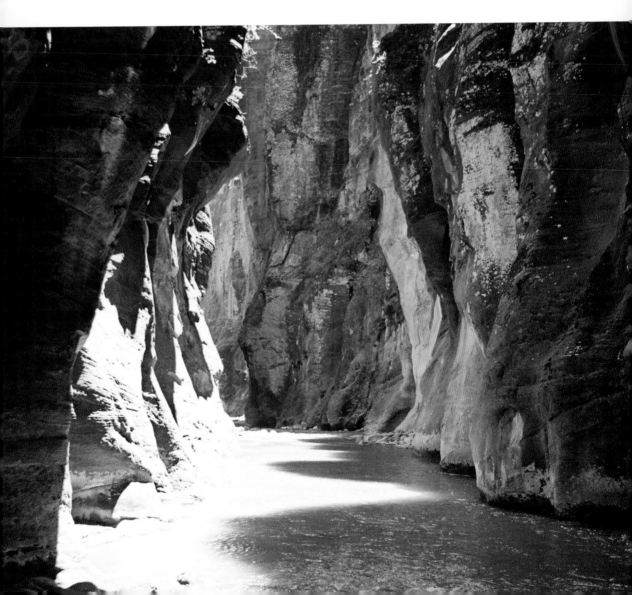

on the lawn of the Zion Lodge at dusk and provide nightly entertainment for guests.

LODGING AND CAMPING

The only lodging inside the park is the historic Zion Lodge. The rustic cabins offered by the lodge are a personal favorite of mine. Reservations at Zion Lodge can be made through Xanterra Parks & Resorts at (888) 297-2757 or at **www.zionlodge.com.** An additional benefit to staying at the lodge is access to the park. Only Zion Lodge guests are permitted to drive into the canyon. Other visitors must use the park shuttle buses that run from April through October. Other lodging options are available outside the south park entrance in Springdale, Utah.

There are two main campgrounds in the park with a total of 340 sites. South Campground is operated on a first-come, first-serve basis, while Watchman Campground takes reservations at **www.recreation .gov.** Campground fees range from $16 to $20 per night.

FEES AND CONTACTS

The park entrance permit is $25 per vehicle for a seven-day pass. Walk-in permits for the Zion Narrows are issued the day of the hike or the day before the hike at the Zion Canyon Backcountry Desk in Zion Canyon Visitor Center. Backcountry Desk hours in the summer are from 7 a.m. to 7 p.m., and permits are $5 per person. Advance reservations for permits can be made online at **www.nps.gov/zion.** Reservations are limited to 40 hikers per day in the Zion Narrows. Weather forecasts, stream reports, and flash flood–potential ratings are all available at the Backcountry Desk, (435) 772-0170. Permits will not be issued when the flow and/or the potential for flash flood are high.

Additional information can be obtained by contacting Zion National Park, Springdale, UT 84767-1099, or by phoning the Zion Canyon Visitor Center at (435) 772-3256. The Park Web site is at **www.nps.gov/zion.**

10 PUEBLO ALTO LOOP

Location: *Chaco Culture National Historic Park, NM*
Distance: *5.3 miles*
Elevation Extremes: *6,110 to 6,450 feet*
Total Elevation Gain: *400 feet*
Difficulty: *Moderate*
USGS Maps: *Pueblo Bonito 7.5-minute*
Trailhead Coordinates: *N 36° 3' 45.3" W 107° 57' 56.6"*
UTM 13S 0232872 3994964 [WSG84]

THE CENTER OF THE ANCIENT WORLD

Getting to Chaco Canyon is not easy. Before my arrival, torrential rains had flooded the high desert of northwestern New Mexico, and I looked across a lake where the road used to be. A four-wheel-drive Jeep had just gone across. Its driver barely pulled it off, and he looked back at me to see what I would do. There was no debate. I shook my head, turned our little rental car around, and headed south back down 20 miles of dirt road toward Navajo Highway 9. Our hike at Chaco Canyon would have to wait until another day.

Two days later my wife, Mary Fran, and I were again headed into Chaco Canyon, this time from the north. Again we were stopped by water on the road, but it was only hubcap deep and we just managed to wallow across. A few minutes later we crossed the boundary into Chaco Cultural National Historic Park and descended into Chaco Canyon. This was once the center of the ancient world in the American Southwest.

The scale and mystery of Chaco are almost impossible to comprehend. Here, in this remote and unforgiving landscape, an ancient people built grand pueblos with a total of 3,000 rooms that reached up to four stories high. Heavy stones were carried from the mesas above, and an estimated 220,000 massive timbers were hauled 50 to 70 miles from distant mountains. The largest structure, Pueblo Bonito, was one of the great creations of the ancient world—as large as the Roman Colosseum. Why did they build these imposing structures in this barren place? Why are there so many dark and forbidding interior rooms with no light or ventilation? And why, after 250 years of arduous construction, did they seal the doorways, burn their kivas (underground ceremonial structures), and move away? Our Chaco Canyon hike would reveal tantalizing clues, but few answers, to these profound mysteries.

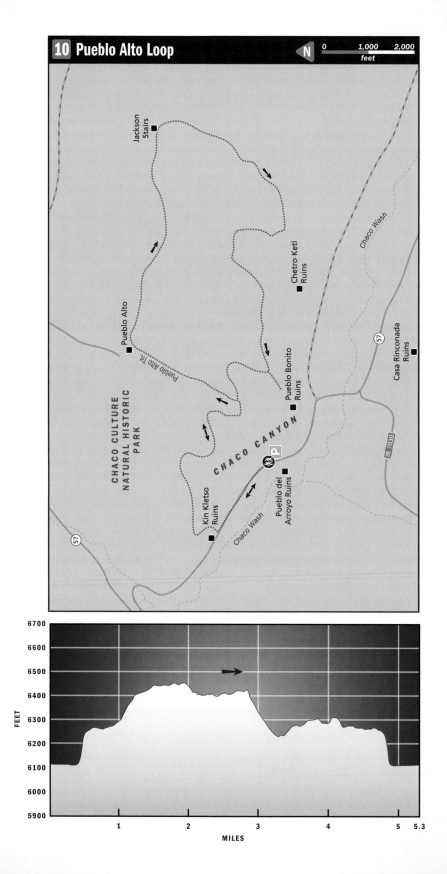

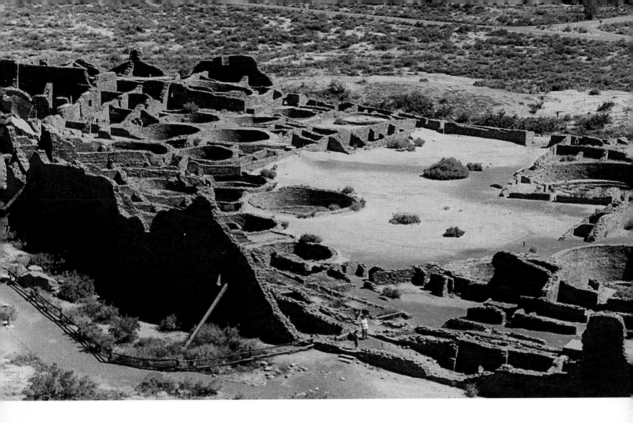

Pueblo Bonito, one of the great structures of the ancient world

Despite recent record rainstorms, it was very hot in Chaco Canyon in the early August of our hike. Mary Fran and I stopped at the visitor center for an introduction to the canyon, and to get a backcountry hiking permit. We then drove west to the Pueblo del Arroyo parking area. There was a picnic table, so we had lunch before setting out. It was during our picnic lunch that I began to realize just how hot it was.

We began hiking after lunch at about 12:45 p.m. We soon came to Kin Kletso, the first of the pueblo ruins along the trail. Like the other great houses at Chaco Canyon, Kin Kletso is an enigma. It originally had more than 100 rooms, five enclosed kivas, and rose three stories high. Curiously, it does not seem to have been intended for residential use, but was rather built to overwhelm and impress.

We found the trailhead for the Pueblo Alto Trail behind Kin Kletso, and started up a steep talus slope and into a narrow fissure in the rock above. This part of the trail was much more difficult than I expected. At times it seemed more like rock climbing than hiking. We struggled up steep steps and over giant blocks of sandstone. Finally, we gained the bench above and turned east on slickrock winding above the box canyons below. Across the canyon we had a good view of Pueblo del Arroyo, an amazing ruin with about 280 rooms and 20 kivas.

We turned left at a trail junction toward Pueblo Alto at about 2 p.m. As we turned uphill, the midday heat—possibly over 100°F—closed in on us. Mary Fran's face was uncommonly red, and I suggested turning back. But she would not be deterred, and we continued on to the top of the mesa.

We soon came to Pueblo Alto, the highest ruin and a very unique complex. Perched on the top of the mesa, the view from Pueblo Alto extends from the La Plata Mountains in southern Colorado to Mount Taylor to the south. Line-on-sight connections can be made with several important locations, including Tsin Kletzin on the mesa across the canyon, a signal station in South Gap, and several pueblos to the north. Pueblo Alto is also the main focal point of 220 miles of prehistoric roads built to link Chaco Canyon to other sites in the Southwest. The Great North Road, which is 30 feet wide, begins at Pueblo Alto and leads 35 miles north to no place in particular. Two days earlier a guide at Acoma Pueblo, the "Sky City," told us that the road north pointed . . . to our point of origin—back to our creator." Even more remarkable, and like most other ruins at Chaco Canyon, the walls of Pueblo Alto were built in exact alignment with the rising of the sun.

After pondering the remains of Pueblo Alto, we continued east across the mesa, past other lesser-known but still outstanding ruins, and down to a viewpoint for the Jackson Stairs. This precarious stairway was built by the Chacoans as an ancient route from the canyon bottom to the top of the mesa. Today it is considered a dangerous passage.

The trail descended the slickrock and continued down through a crack to a lower bench with a good view of Chetro Ketl, one of the largest Chacoan structures. The builders of Chetro Ketl constructed an immense elevated plaza that rises above the surrounding landscape. An estimated 500 rooms and 16 kivas, including a huge "great kiva," surrounded the plaza.

Finally we made our way to a point where a side trail led down to a viewpoint overlooking Pueblo Bonito. By traveling the loop trail clockwise, the best was saved for last. Mary Fran, however, was feeling the combined effects of heat and altitude, and elected to continue down toward the trailhead. I walked to the Pueblo Bonito viewpoint and was awestruck. It is an immense D-shaped complex with walls perfectly aligned to the rising of the sun. This gigantic edifice, itself considered the center of the Chacoan world, towered four stories high and contained more than 600 rooms and 40 kivas. Here again, the structure itself does not seem constructed for residential use. There are few burial sites in the canyon, and the refuse dumps are not characteristic of domestic use.

A short time later I rejoined Mary Fran; we headed back down the narrow fissure in the rock, past Kin Kletso, and were back at the trailhead at the Pueblo del Arroyo parking area by 4:30 p.m. We were both tired and parched from the sun, but this memory would last a lifetime. Nothing quite like Chaco Canyon, the "center of the ancient world," has existed before or since.

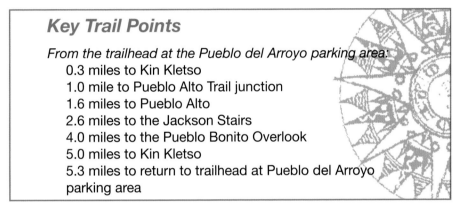

Key Trail Points

From the trailhead at the Pueblo del Arroyo parking area:
- 0.3 miles to Kin Kletso
- 1.0 mile to Pueblo Alto Trail junction
- 1.6 miles to Pueblo Alto
- 2.6 miles to the Jackson Stairs
- 4.0 miles to the Pueblo Bonito Overlook
- 5.0 miles to Kin Kletso
- 5.3 miles to return to trailhead at Pueblo del Arroyo parking area

DIRECTIONS TO TRAILHEAD AND TRAIL ROUTE

Chaco Canyon lies in isolated beauty in the high desert of northwestern New Mexico. The recommended access route is from the north. Turn off US 550 3 miles east of Nageezi, or about 50 miles west of Cuba, onto County Road 7900. Follow CR 7900 and 7950 south on a paved surface for 5 miles, and an additional 16 miles on a dirt surface to the park boundary. Access from the south takes even longer over rough dirt roads. From the south, turn north from Interstate 40 at Thoreau on New Mexico 371. After 24 miles, turn east on CR 9 to Seven Lakes. At Seven Lakes, turn north on NM 57 and travel 20 miles over rough dirt to the park.

Once in the park, stop at the visitor center for a free backcountry hiking permit. From the visitor center, drive west on the paved park road for 4.5 miles to the Pueblo del Arroyo parking area. Walk west past a gate on an old dirt road to Kin Kletso. A sign directly behind Kin Kletso marks the beginning of the Pueblo Alto Trail. Follow the trail winding up the talus slope to a narrow crack through the rock, and onto the first bench on the mesa above. Turn left at a trail junction 0.7 miles from Kin Kletso toward Pueblo Alto. This loop trail then leads to Pueblo Alto, across the mesa top and down slickrock to the top of the Jackson Stairs. The trail then runs south along a mesa top, down through a narrow crack, and then down to the first bench above the canyon. The trail follows this bench back to the Pueblo Alto Trail junction, skirting box canyons along the way. From the trail junction, descend back down through the narrow crack above Kin Kletso, and follow the old dirt road back to the Pueblo del Arroyo parking area.

WEATHER AND WILDLIFE

The weather in Chaco Canyon in unpredictable and can be extreme. Summer temperatures are typically in the 80s to mid-90s, but can reach 110°F. When hiking, be sure to take plenty of water and protection from the sun. There is no shade on the Pueblo Alto Trail. Winter temperatures are commonly below freezing. Spring and fall offer more moderate temperatures.

A herd of 50 to 60 elk migrated into the park in 2000 and can still be seen in the canyon along with deer and pronghorn antelope. Leashed pets are permitted on trails, but are not allowed to enter the cultural sites.

LODGING AND CAMPING

Lodging can be found north of the park along US 550. A small campground is located 1 mile east of the visitor center. Camping is $10 per night on a first-come, first-serve basis. At press time, the campground was reduced to only 35 sites due to emergency repairs because of flood damage.

FEES AND CONTACTS

The entrance fee is $8 per vehicle for a seven-day pass, and the park is open all year.

For more information write Chaco Culture National Historic Park, PO Box 220, Nageezi, NM 87037, or phone (505) 786-7014. The park Web site is **www.nps.gov/chcu.**

Kin Kletso from the Pueblo Alto Trail

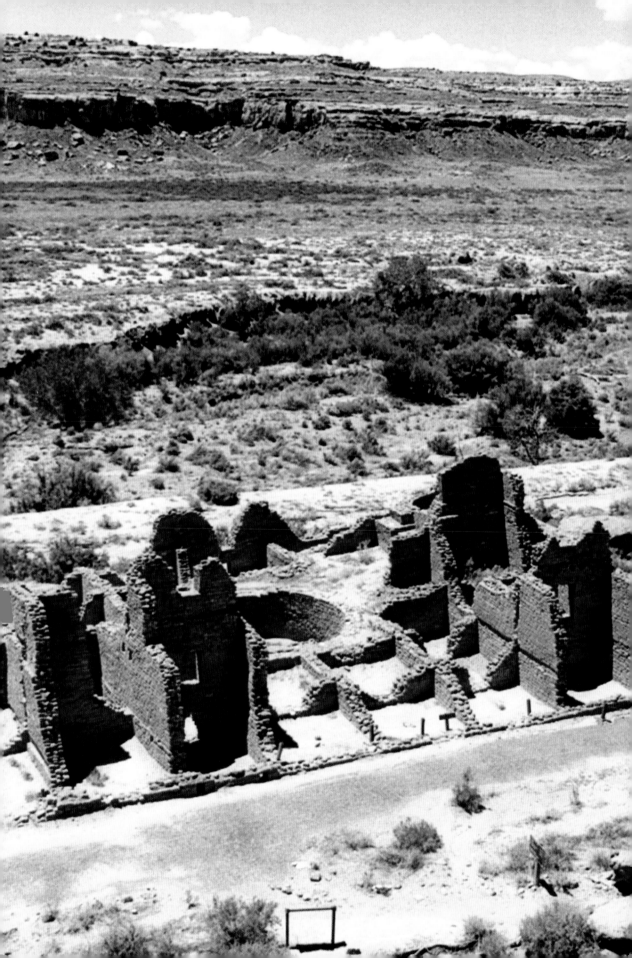

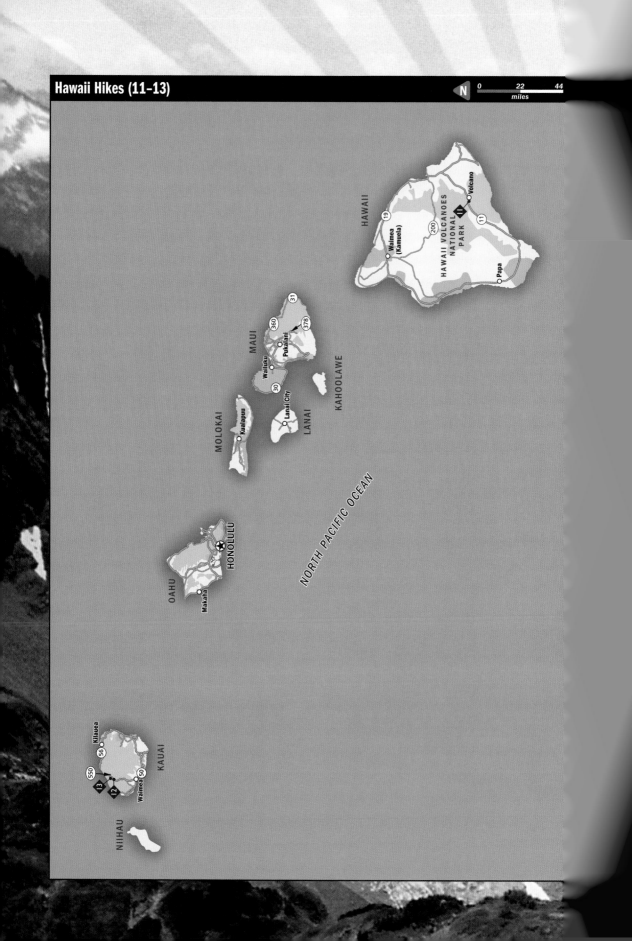

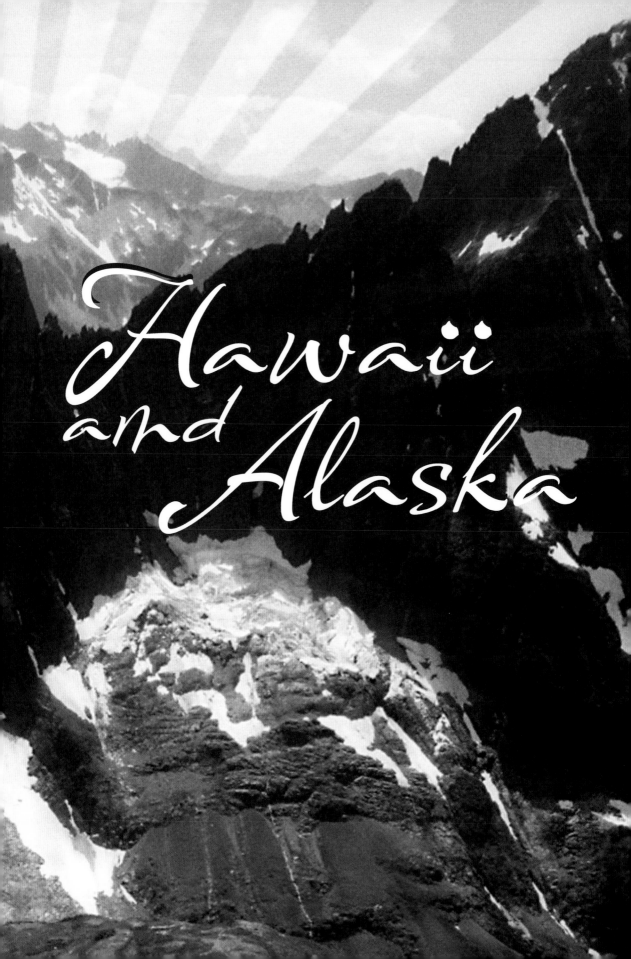

Hawaii and Alaska

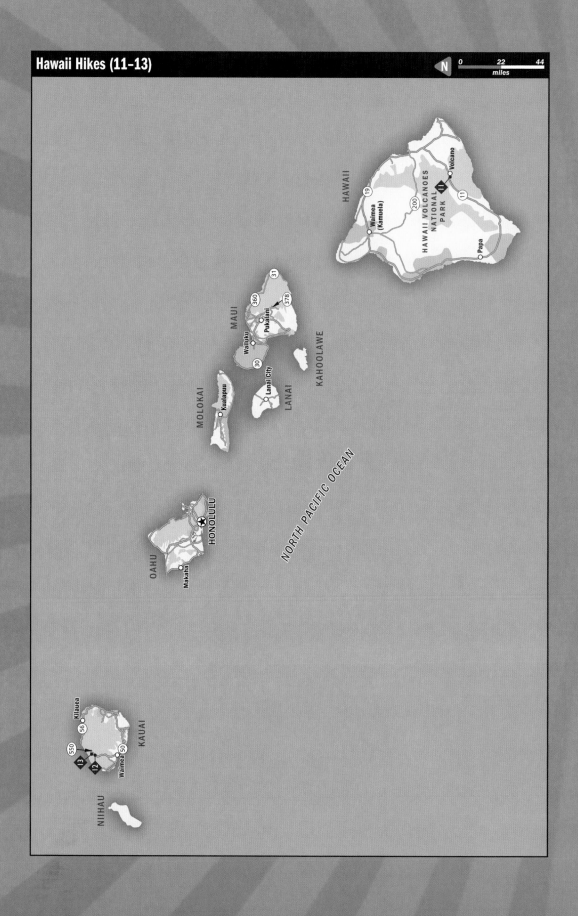

N

0   22   44
miles

NORTH PACIFIC OCEAN

HAWAII

⑲

⑳⓪

⑪

Waimea
(Kamuela)

HAWAII VOLCANOES
NATIONAL
PARK

Volcano

Papa

MAUI

㉛

㊱⓪

378

Pukalani

Wailuku

㉚

KAHOOLAWE

MOLOKAI

Kualapuu

Lanai City

LANAI

HONOLULU

OAHU

Makaha

NIIHAU

Kilauea

㊺

550

13

12

Waimea

㊿

KAUAI

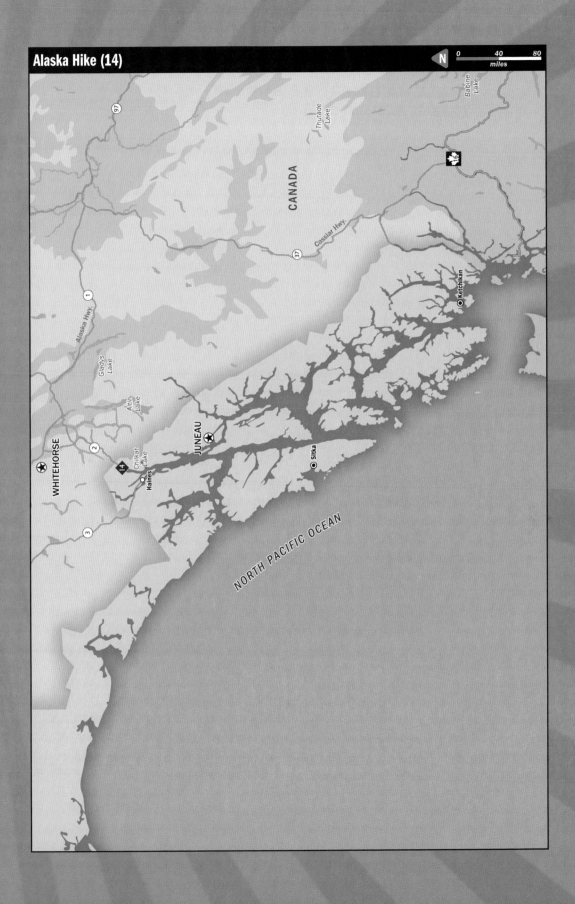

11 KILAUEA VOLCANO
(HALEMA'UMA'U, KILAUEA IKI, AND CRATER RIM TRAILS)

Location: *Hawaii Volcanoes National Park, HI*
Distance: *9.6 miles*
Elevation Extremes: *3,540 feet to 3,970 feet*
Total Elevation Gain: *800 feet*
Difficulty: *Strenuous*
USGS Maps: *Kilauea Crater 7.5-minute, Volcano 7.5-minute*
Trailhead Coordinates: *N 19° 25' 42.0" W 155° 15' 29.0"*
                            UTM 5Q 0262890 2149770 [WGS 84]

THE HOUSE OF PELE

Nothing can quite compare to your first view of the smoldering Kilauea Crater. The floor of the massive crater is starkly barren, with steam and volcanic gases rising from the underworld below. It appears to be a sight from Hades. Improbable as it seemed, we planned to hike directly across the floor of the smoking crater before us.

Most volcanoes and earthquakes occur at the edges of the earth's tectonic plates, as adjoining plates collide or grind against one another. But the Hawaiian volcanoes are different. They are fueled by a massive hot spot in the earth's mantle, about 60 miles beneath the floor of the sea. For 70 million years, molten rock rising from the hot spot has created a long series of volcanoes as the Pacific Plate drifted overhead at a rate of about four inches per year. Kilauea Volcano is currently located directly above this hot spot.

Nearly as remarkable as the crater itself is the surprise of finding a good hotel at the edge of an active volcano. The dining room of the historic Volcano House looks out on the scene, and houseguests have often been treated to pyrotechnics along with their dinner. My family and I had come to Hawaii for the annual Highpointers Club convention, and also for the unmatched hiking opportunities that Hawaii has to offer. The day before visiting Kilauea Crater, we had walked to the top of Mauna Kea, which is the highest point in Hawaii at 13,796 feet. There we met Henri Butler, who, with his ascent to Mauna Kea, had just completed his travels to the highest points in all 50 states. Henri wanted to join me on this classic hike across Kilauea Crater. My wife and daughter—Mary Fran and Jenny—would be driving to meet us

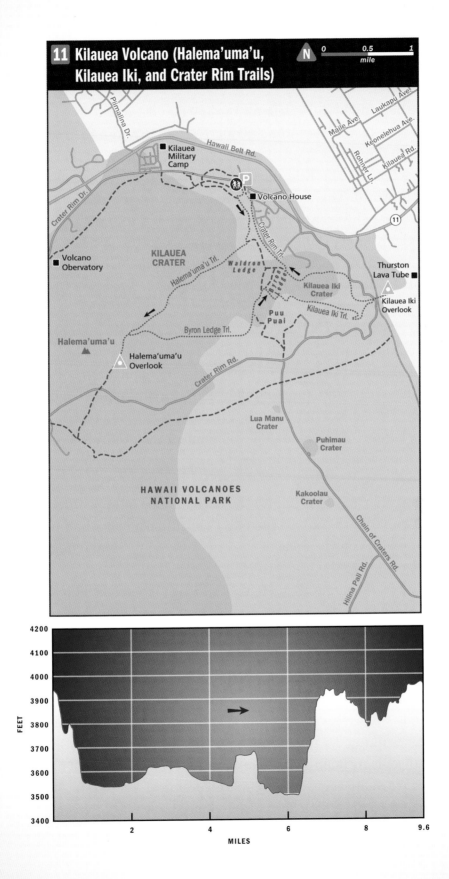

11 Kilauea Volcano (Halema'uma'u, Kilauea Iki, and Crater Rim Trails)

N

0   0.5   1
mile

Piimalina Dr.

Laukapu Ave.

Maile Ave.

Keonelehua Ave.

Rohier Ln.

Kilauea Rd.

Hawaii Belt Rd.

Kilauea Military Camp

P

Volcano House

11

Crater Rim Dr.

Crater Rim Trl.

Volcano Obervatory

KILAUEA CRATER

Halema'uma'u Trl.

Waldron Ledge

Byron Ledge

Kilauea Iki Crater

Thurston Lava Tube

Kilauea Iki Overlook

Kilauea Iki Trl.

Puu Puai

Byron Ledge Trl.

Halema'uma'u

Halema'uma'u Overlook

Crater Rim Rd.

Lua Manu Crater

Puhimau Crater

HAWAII VOLCANOES NATIONAL PARK

Kakoolau Crater

Chain of Craters Rd.

Hilina Pali Rd.

4200
4100
4000
3900
3800
3700
3600
3500
3400

FEET

2   4   6   8   9.6

MILES

along the way. We pulled up to the Volcano House Hotel midmorning and located the start of the Halema'uma'u Trail directly behind the dining room.

From the trailhead, Henri and I proceeded 0.4 miles down the Halema'uma'u Trail, descending about 400 feet through lush tropical vegetation to the crater floor. Here the jungle gave way to the stark, barren lava flows of the Kilauea Crater. It was as if we had stepped into another world. The passage of the trail across the hard, black lava was marked only by occasional cairns constructed to show the way. Although the Kilauea Caldera itself has not been the site of a major eruption since 1952, its central crater, Halema'uma'u, has been the site of intermittent activity, and lava flows have flooded parts of the caldera floor as recently as 1982.

We arrived at the Halema'uma'u Overlook at 10:45 a.m. to meet Mary Fran and Jenny, who had taken Crater Rim Drive. The central pit of Halema'uma'u Crater is an extraordinary sight! It is 250 feet deep, 1 mile across, and punctuated by sulphureous smoke and fumes. The ancient Hawaiians believed that the goddess Pele made her home in Kilauea Crater. The jealous Pele demanded tribute from her subjects, and sometimes paid them terrifying visits through her subterranean passageways. When threatened by eruptions, frightened Hawaiians cast offerings of pigs into the lava in hope of appealing Pele's wrath. Hawaiians still pay homage to Pele, and someone had placed several flower leis on the edge of the crater, possibly in an effort to appease the goddess of the underworld.

After a few moments rest, Henri and I turned our back on Halema'uma'u and retraced our steps 0.4 miles to Byron Ledge Trail. We followed Byron Ledge Trail across the Kilauea Caldera and up Byron Ledge to Kilauea Iki Trail. From here we dropped into Kilauea Iki Crater. Kilauea Iki, meaning "little Kilauea," was the site of a massive eruption in 1959. Although it is smaller than the main crater, it is actually more impressive, with its steep walls and still-steaming lava flows. After walking 2.4 miles across the floor of Kilauea Iki Crater, we climbed 400 feet through native rain forest to the Lava Tube parking area. Here we again met Mary Fran and Jenny at 12:40 p.m. It had taken me and Henri a little over three hours to arrive at this point, having covered a total of 7.4 incredible miles.

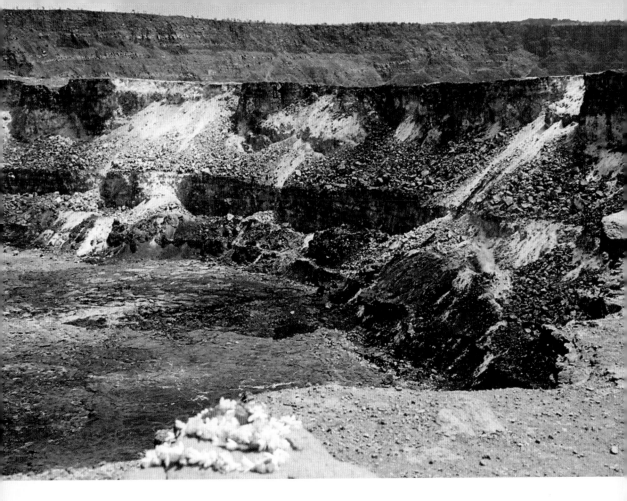

Halama'uma'u Crater with an offering to Pele

We took a welcome break at the Lava Tube parking area for
lunch and to explore the Thurston Lava Tube. A well-traveled asphalt trail led into the tube, and electric lighting lit the tunnel for
the first few hundred feet. Beyond that, the trail emerged back into
the rain forest. We brought flashlights and explored the lava tube a
short distance beyond the electric lights, but lava tubes are relatively
uninteresting compared with their limestone counterparts. There are
no flowstone formations and they lack complexity, being essentially
long subway-like tunnels that drained out when the source of lava
ceased to flow. So after a few minutes we turned our attention back to
the trail.

From the Lava Tube parking area, Crater Rim Trail led 0.5 miles to
Kilauea Iki Overlook, and finally another 1.7 miles back to the Volcano
House Hotel. This final remarkable stretch of trail had some of the best
views of the day. Our brief glimpse into the fiery house of Pele was as
unique and spellbinding as any experience I have known.

Key Trail Points

From the trailhead behind Volcano House Hotel:
- 0.4 miles to the Kilauea Crater floor
- 2.6 miles to Halema'uma'u Overlook
- 5.0 miles to Kilauea Iki Trail
- 7.4 miles to Thurston Lava Tube parking area
- 7.9 miles to Kilauea Iki Overlook
- 9.6 miles to return to the trailhead behind Volcano House

DIRECTIONS TO TRAILHEAD AND TRAIL ROUTE

To reach Hawaii Volcanoes National Park, drive 27 miles south from Hilo, Hawaii, on HI 11. The entrance station to the park is located just off HI 11 on Crater Rim Drive, and the Volcano House Hotel is 0.3 miles west of the entrance station.

Kilauea Crater from Volcano House

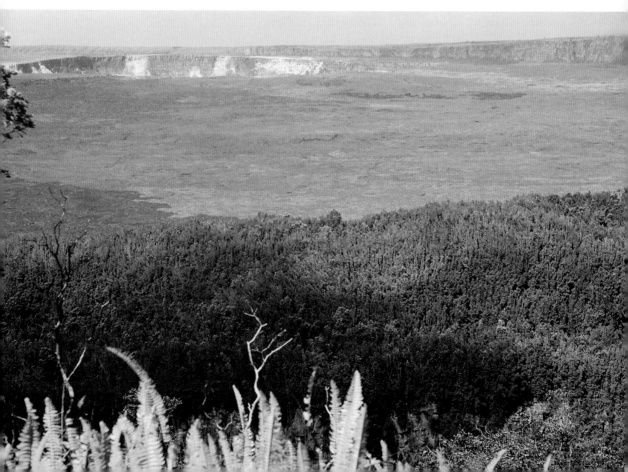

From the Halema'uma'u trailhead, behind Volcano House, descend Halema'uma'u Trail about 400 feet to the floor of Kilauea Caldera and cross the caldera to Halema'uma'u Overlook at the central crater. This part of the trail is not without risk. The cairns that mark the location of the trail are not always obvious, and some care is needed to stay on route. Lava crusts and cliffs are often unstable, and falling on sharp lava can inflict serious wounds. Furthermore, volcanic fumes may be encountered, particularly near Halema'uma'u Crater, which can be hazardous to persons with respiratory problems.

From Halema'uma'u Overlook, backtrack 0.4 miles on Halema'uma'u Trail to Byron Ledge Trail. Turn right onto Byron Ledge Trail and continue 1.5 miles across Kilauea Crater, then 0.5 miles up Byron Ledge to Kilauea Iki Trail. Turn right onto Kilauea Iki Trail, walk across the steaming floor of Kilauea Iki Crater, and climb about 400 feet to the Thurston Lava Tube parking area. Take time to explore this interesting cave formed by flowing lava.

Cross the Lava Tube parking area and locate Crater Rim Trail leading to Kilauea Iki Overlook. Continue west on Crater Rim Trail 1.7 miles back to the trailhead at the Volcano House Hotel.

WEATHER AND WILDLIFE

The weather in Hawaii Volcanoes National Park is highly changeable, and can be rainy and chilly at the crater rim any time of year.

Hikers are not likely to encounter wildlife in or near Kilauea Crater, except for birds and bats near dusk. With luck, hikers may glimpse the nene, a rare and treasured Hawaiian goose that looks like a Canada goose with zebra stripes. I encountered nene on a hike in Haleakala National Park on Maui when I paused for lunch. I actually had to push one away when he made a lunge for my sandwich. He expressed his displeasure by honking at me, and made another attempt for my sandwich. This time, a thump on the head finally convinced him to feed elsewhere—so much for the shy and elusive nene. Feeding them encourages the birds to beg, and endangers their lives.

LODGING AND CAMPING

The only lodging inside the park is the Volcano House Hotel located on the northern edge of the crater. I stayed at Volcano House in 1985 and highly recommend it for an unforgettable experience. Reservations should be made early at (808) 967-7321 or **www.volcanohousehotel .com.** Bed-and-breakfast accommodations, as well as other services, can be found in Volcano Village located 1 mile east of the park.

The park has two drive-in campgrounds. Namakanipaio is located off HI 11 3 miles west of the entrance station. Kulanaokuaiki Campground is located 5 miles down the Hilina Pali Road and has no water. Camping is free of charge and available on a first-come, first-served basis. Volcano House Hotel also operates rustic camper cabins at the Namakanipaio Campground; reservations are required.

FEES AND CONTACTS

The entrance fee for the park is $10 per vehicle or $5 per individual for a seven-day pass.

Current information is available by writing the Superintendent, Hawaii Volcanoes National Park, PO Box 52, Hawaii National Park, HI 96718-0052, or visit the park Web site at **www.nps.gov/havo.** For an update on current volcanic activity, phone (808) 985-6000 day or night.

Trail to the Thurston Lava Tube

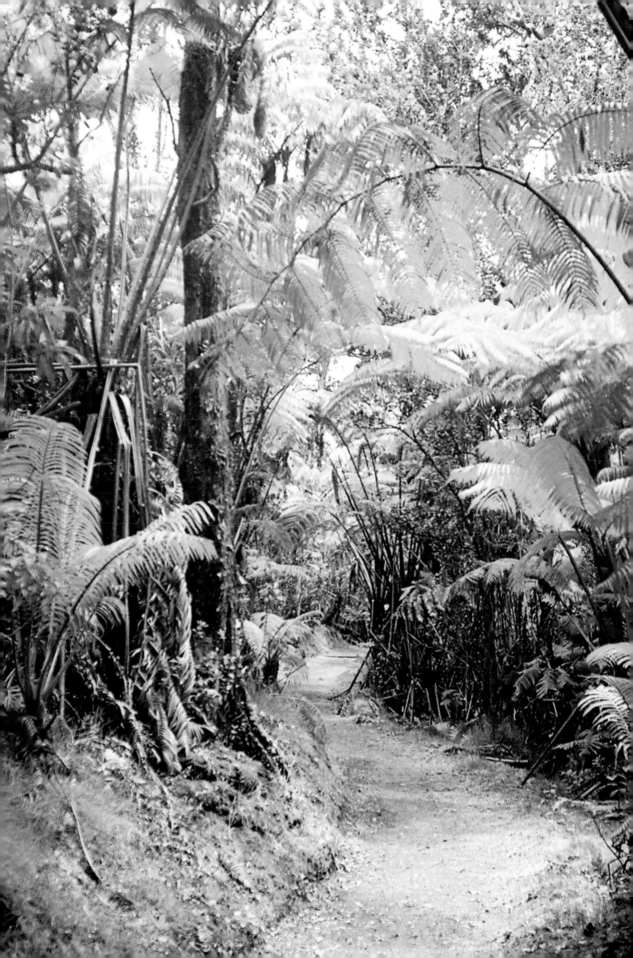

12 WAIMEA CANYON LOOP
(CANYON, KUMUWELA, AND HALEMANU TRAILS)

Location: *Koke'e State Park, Kauai, HI*
Distance: *7.2 miles*
Elevation Extremes: *3,200 feet to 3,810 feet*
Total Elevation Gain: *1,080 feet*
Difficulty: *Moderate*
USGS Maps: *Makaha Point 7.5-minute, Waimea Canyon 7.5-minute, Haena 7.5-minute*
Trailhead Coordinates: *N 22° 6' 56.0" W 159° 40' 9.4"*

THE GRAND CANYON OF THE PACIFIC

Hawaiian legend tells us that this land was born from the fiery fury of Pele, the volcano goddess, who left Kauai after failing to find a suitable home. As she leaped eastward to the neighboring island of Oahu, Pele left her footprint atop the rim of Kauai's Waimea Canyon.

Mark Twain first christened this remarkable chasm the "Grand Canyon of the Pacific." Waimea Canyon is much younger than its 200 million-year-old counterpart in Arizona, but it does bear a striking resemblance. The canyon owes its exceptional beauty to 10 million years of erosion, which changed the landscape and shaped the dormant volcanoes into jagged peaks and deep canyons. Today Waimea Canyon is 1 mile wide, more than 10 miles long, and over 3,000 feet deep. It is a mecca for hikers and sightseers who marvel as shadows of clouds and changing light paint the canyon walls.

Including a Waimea Canyon hike in my plan was easy, but choosing the exact hike was a problem. This magnificent canyon is laced with trails, and each offers its own unique brand of enchantment. From the early research I had done, my first candidate was Kukui Trail, which drops steeply all the way to the canyon floor. But on the strong advice of the Koke'e State Park rangers, I switched my plans to a loop including Canyon Trail and beautiful Waipoo Falls.

On a late morning in August, my family and I left our parked rental car at the top of Halemanu Road and hiked steeply down the road to the Canyon Trail–Black Pipe Trail junction. After a short side trip down Cliff Trail to a lovely canyon lookout, we continued down Canyon Trail to an exposed knoll with beautiful open views of the canyon. A trail to the right

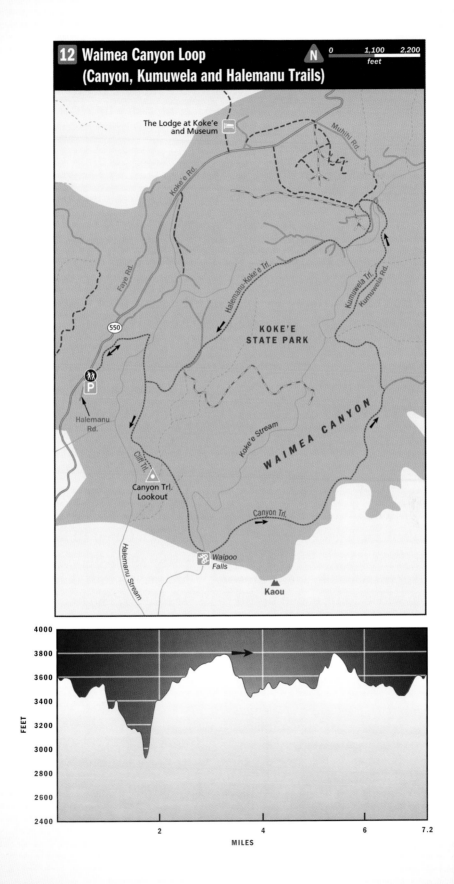

12 **Waimea Canyon Loop**
(Canyon, Kumuwela and Halemanu Trails)

N   0   1,100   2,200
feet

The Lodge at Koke'e
and Museum

Muhihi Rd.

Koke'e Rd.

Faye Rd.

Halemanu-Koke'e Trl.

Kumuwela Trl.

Kumuwela Rd.

550

KOKE'E
STATE PARK

Halemanu
Rd.

Cliff Trl.

Koke'e Stream

WAIMEA CANYON

Canyon Trl.
Lookout

Canyon Trl.

Halemanu Stream

Waipoo
Falls

Kaou

FEET

4000
3800
3600
3400
3200
3000
2800
2600
2400

2   4   6   7.2
MILES

then brought us to the brink of the two-tiered 800-foot Waipoo Falls. Pools where people swim were perched at the very brink of the lower falls, which plunged vertically 600 feet into the canyon. It was 12:40 p.m., and this cool oasis seemed like a perfect place for lunch.

After lunch, my wife and daughter, Mary Fran and Jenny, retraced their steps back to the car, while I crossed Koke'e Stream and continued up Canyon Trail on the far side. This section of trail was crowned with magnificent views hundreds of feet down into Waimea and Po'omau canyons. I reached Kumuwela Road at 2 p.m., after climbing about 600 feet above the falls. Continuing north, I spotted Kumuwela Trail. It was fainter and obviously less traveled than Canyon Trail, but it too had its own special magic. Kumuwela Trail meandered steeply up and down in a vine-covered jungle, and was completely different from the canyon-rim trails. More than 460 inches of annual rainfall have transformed this jungle into an alien world where few foreign plants and animals have invaded. Cattle and goats destroyed much of the ancient Hawaiian habitat, and nonnative birds introduced to the island carried mosquito-born diseases that decimated native bird populations. But the jungle atop Kauai, being too high for mosquitoes and largely untouched by feral animals, is the last refuge for a host of native Hawaiian plants and birds, including the last o'o a'a, the rarest bird in the world.

I reached a four-wheel-drive road at 2:20 p.m., which I followed to Camp 10 Road to return to Koke'e Lodge and Museum. After a short break at the lodge, I retraced my steps down Camp 10 Road to Halemanu-Koke'e Trail. I followed this easy trail through fragrant koa jungle, blackberry patches, and crowing wild roosters to Halemanu Road, from which I proceeded uphill to the trailhead. The hike was a splendid mix of spectacular canyon vistas, a dramatic 800-foot waterfall, and fragrant tropical jungles.

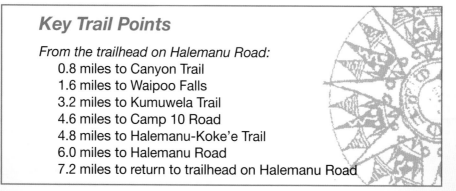

Key Trail Points

From the trailhead on Halemanu Road:
- 0.8 miles to Canyon Trail
- 1.6 miles to Waipoo Falls
- 3.2 miles to Kumuwela Trail
- 4.6 miles to Camp 10 Road
- 4.8 miles to Halemanu-Koke'e Trail
- 6.0 miles to Halemanu Road
- 7.2 miles to return to trailhead on Halemanu Road

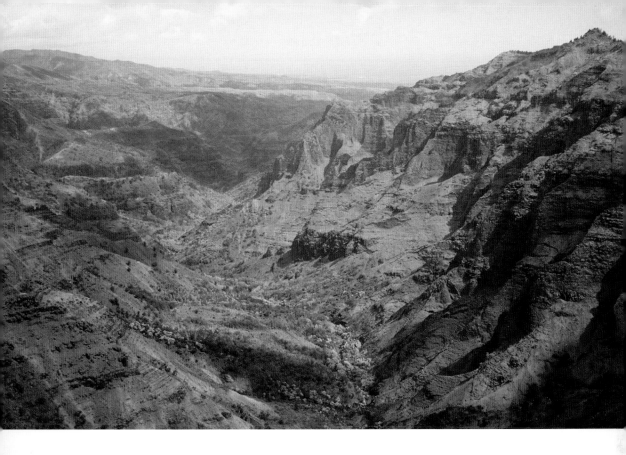

Waimea Canyon, the "Grand Canyon of the Pacific"

DIRECTIONS TO TRAILHEAD AND TRAIL ROUTE

To reach Koke'e State Park and Waimea Canyon, turn up Waimea
Canyon Drive/HI 550 at Waimea Town. This approach is narrow and
rougher than the road above Kekaha, but is much more scenic. Waimea
Canyon Drive merges with Koke'e Road after a few miles. Continue on
HI 550 to the Koke'e Lodge and Museum. Check for trail and road con-
ditions at the Division of State Parks office before proceeding.

To begin the hike, retrace HI 550 south from Koke'e Lodge 1.4
miles to Halemanu Road, a four-wheel-drive track. Parking is available
on both sides of the road. Hike down Halemanu Road 0.8 miles to the
trailhead marked Canyon and Black Pipe trails. About 100 yards down
the trail is Cliff Trail, a short spur to a beautiful canyon overlook. After
admiring the view, return to Canyon Trail and continue down past the
Black Pipe Trail junction; Canyon Trail then bears right and levels out
onto a large bare knoll overlooking the canyon. From the lower edge of
the knoll the trail veers left down to Koke'e Stream and Waipoo Falls.
Waipoo is a two-tiered 800-foot waterfall, and is worth every step that
it takes to get there. At this point you have dropped 600 feet in 1.6
miles from the parking area.

Cross Koke'e Stream and climb Canyon Trail 600 feet in 1.2 miles to Kumuwela Road, another four-wheel-drive track. This section of trail has magnificent, open views of the canyon. Continue on Kumuwela Road about 0.4 miles, then turn left on Kumuwela Trail. Continue 0.8 miles to the end of the trail at a four-wheel-drive road in a private camp. Follow the rough road 0.6 miles uphill, then turn left on Camp 10 Road to the Koke'e Lodge and Museum. Total distance from the parking lot to the museum is 5.2 miles.

To close the loop, after traveling only 0.1 mile on Camp 10 Road, turn left onto a road posted with a "Camp Sloggett" sign. Continue on this road 0.1 mile to an old ranger station, and then turn right at the Halemanu-Koke'e Trailhead. Follow the Halemanu-Koke'e Trail to Halemanu Road. Join Halemanu Road and continue about 0.4 miles to the junction with Canyon Trail, then retrace the inbound route 0.8 miles uphill to the parking lot.

Waimea Canyon from Cliff Trail Overlook

WEATHER AND WILDLIFE

Temperatures in the jungle atop Kauai average a cool 60°F, providing a welcome change in climate from the lower elevations, particularly in summer. The windchill factor can drop into the 40s even in summer, while winter temperatures drop into the 30s overnight. This is one of the wettest places on earth, so bring raingear, especially during the tradewinds. During periods of heavy rain, stream crossings may be hazardous. Although there is an abundance of water in the jungle, it is not fit for drinking, so bring your own. Weather in the open canyon is somewhat drier and warmer.

The jungle of Kauai is the last refuge of several rare Hawaiian birds. The white-tailed Tropicbird, an elegant soaring bird with a two-foot wingspan, comes to Kauai to lay its eggs and can also be seen gracing the walls of the canyon. Unfortunately, other common "wildlife" seen on this hike are feral chickens and roosters.

LODGING AND CAMPING

Cabins equipped with hot showers, kitchen facilities, and fireplaces can be rented from The Lodge at Koke'e for $35–$45 per night. A broader range of services and lodging can be found 19 miles south along HI 50.

Koke'e offers four campgrounds, one in Koke'e State Park on HI 550 and three primitive Division of Forestry campgrounds along Camp 10 Road. Depending on conditions, the latter three may require four-wheel-drive vehicles to reach them. Permits are required for all campsites, and can be applied for at park headquarters near The Lodge at Koke'e.

FEES AND CONTACTS

There is no entrance or parking fee for Koke'e State Park. Cabin and campsite permits can be arranged from The Lodge at Koke'e at PO Box 367, Waimea, HI 96796, online at **www.thelodgeatkokee.net,** or by phone at (808) 335-6061. Additional information regarding trails and local conditions can be obtained from the Division of State Parks at 3060 Eiwa Street, #306, Lihue, HI 96766-1875, online at **www .hawaiistateparks.org/parks/kauai,** or by phone at (808) 274-3444.

13 KALALAU TRAIL

Location: *Na Pali Coast, Kauai, HI*
Distance: *13 miles (to Hanakoa and return)*
Elevation Extremes: *20 feet to 780 feet*
Total Elevation Gain: *2,750 feet*
Difficulty: *Very Strenuous*
USGS Maps: *Haena 7.5-minute*
Trailhead Coordinates: *N 22° 13' 13.0" W 159° 34' 59.8"*
UTM 4Q 0439900 2457330

THE MOST BEAUTIFUL COAST IN THE WORLD

Once you've experienced the Na Pali Coast on the island of Hawaii, it's easy to see why this soaring cliff has earned the superlative reputation among all who see it. Most agree that it is simply the most beautiful place in Hawaii, and few people that have ever hiked the extraordinary Kalalau Trail would argue the point. Here breath-taking pali, or cliffs, rise abruptly out of an emerald green ocean. Towering waterfalls cascade down sheer gorges, adding to one of the most incredible scenes that nature has ever created. Occasional beaches, appearing as small ribbons of sand, break the imposing majesty of the pali. Kalalau Trail, originally built in the late 1800s, follows the line of an ancient Hawaiian footpath that once linked the remote valleys of the Na Pali Coast.

It was a Sunday in early August, our last full day in Hawaii, and this was what I had been waiting for, the famed Kalalau Trail of the Na Pali Coast. Just two days earlier, high in Koke'e State Park, we had marveled at the fluted cliffs of the Kalalau Valley rising like a turreted emerald castle from the sea 4,000 feet below. At the time, I wondered if I would have the stamina to hike the entire trail to Kalalau Beach and return—a total of 22 grueling miles. My day-use permit extended only to Hanakoa Valley, but I was hoping to push at least a little farther.

My wife and daughter—Mary Fran and Jenny—planned to hike with me the first 2 miles to Hanakapi'ai Beach and return. It was Mary Fran's birthday; she was also anxious to see the cliffs of the Na Pali Coast. We started from the trailhead at Ke'e Beach at about 9:30 a.m., later than I had hoped. The first 2 miles of the trail do not require a permit, and it was crowded with day-hikers as we climbed nearly 600 feet to our first spectacular view of the coast. It was 11 a.m. when we reached Hanakapi'ai Valley, and I was getting anxious to leave civilization behind.

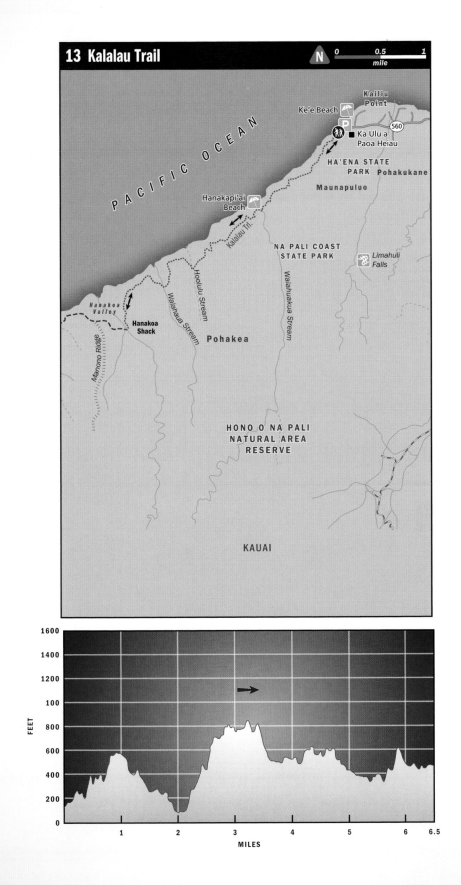

13 Kalalau Trail

N

0   0.5   1
mile

PACIFIC OCEAN

Kailiu Point

Ke'e Beach

Ka Ulu a Paoa Heiau

560

HA'ENA STATE PARK Pohakukane

Maunapuluo

Hanakapi'ai Beach

Kalalau Trl.

NA PALI COAST STATE PARK

Limahuli Falls

Hanakoa Valley

Hanakoa Shack

Hoolulu Stream

Waiahuakua Stream

Waiahaua Stream

Manono Ridge

Pohakea

HONO O NA PALI NATURAL AREA RESERVE

KAUAI

1600
1400
1200
100
800
600
400
200
0

FEET

1   2   3   4   5   6   6.5

MILES

After saying goodbye to Mary Fran and Jenny, I started up the steep switchbacks that climb 800 feet above Hanakapi'ai Beach. The midday tropical heat was already taking a toll on me, and I again regretted not getting an earlier start. The trail climbed higher up the cliffs, traversing the Hono O Na Pali Natural Area Reserve and the dramatic hanging valleys of Ho'olulu and Waiahuakua. The trail seemed to become more spectacular with each passing mile. Two feral goats briefly paused to regard me an instant before disappearing over the sheer cliffs below. I had hoped to average at least 2.5, perhaps even 3, miles per hour, but the steepness of the terrain and the rugged nature of the trail had slowed me to no more than 2 miles per hour.

I finally reached Hanakoa Valley at about 1 p.m. and crossed Hanakoa Stream, determined to press on. But by the time I reached the steep sea cliffs beyond Hanakoa Valley, about 7 miles from the trailhead, it was plainly time to sit down and have a talk with myself. It was nearly 1:30

Secluded beach along the Na Pali Coast

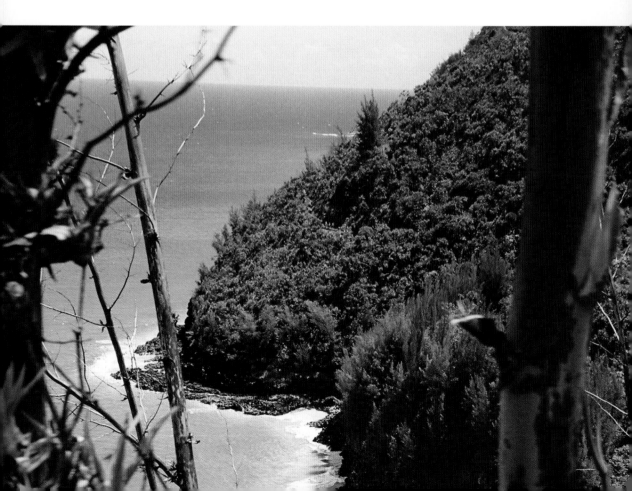

p.m. A panoramic view of the fabled Pali of the Kalalau Valley was urging me on. Would I have the energy to continue on another 3.5 miles to Kalalau Stream, and then return all the way back to Ke'e Beach? Maybe, but I clearly didn't have enough daylight. At the pace I was hiking, I calculated that I would be in total darkness 3 to 4 miles from the trailhead. Mary Fran would probably launch an embarrassing rescue effort, possibly with good reason. It was time to turn back, but the portion of the trail I had already seen could not have been more memorable.

Back at Hanakoa Valley, I stopped for a late lunch. This little island of civilization had a few picnic tables and a small campground. The campsites are on old agricultural terraces where coffee plants, introduced in the late 1800s, are still growing. It was a welcome rest before the long trip back to Ke'e Beach and Mary Fran. As the late afternoon and evening wore on in the tropical heat, my weariness only confirmed the wisdom of turning back when I did. I was learning that the Kalalau Trail was much more demanding than one would expect, based simply on its distance and elevation gain. Fortunately, a couple of quick rain showers helped cool me off. I finally arrived back at the trailhead at about 6:30 p.m., footsore and completely drained. I had a new appreciation for not only the exquisite beauty of the wild and inviolate Na Pali Coast, but also for the unique and arduous character of Kalalau Trail. I had high expectations of the trail, and it did not disappoint me.

Key Trail Points

From the trailhead at Ke'e Beach:
 2.0 miles to Hanakapi'ai Beach
 4.0 miles to Ho'olulu Stream
 6.5 miles to Hanakoa Valley
 13.0 miles to return to the trailhead at Ke'e Beach

DIRECTIONS TO TRAILHEAD AND TRAIL ROUTE

To reach the trailhead, drive north from Lihue on HI 56 on the island of Kauai. Continue on HI 56 and then HI 560 to the end of the road 41 miles from Lihue. The trailhead is at the south end of a large parking area at Ke'e Beach in Ha'ena\ State Park.

Kalalau Trail is well maintained but still very rugged. The path is almost never level, constantly dropping to narrow beaches, then rising hundreds of feet to skirt towering cliffs that drop abruptly into the sea.

Until a few years ago, it was possible to ride a Zodiac raft to Kalalau Beach and walk the trail back to Ke'e Beach. But following the closure of the trail for six months in 1996 due to erosion and unsafe conditions, the Hawaii State Department of Land and Natural Resources adopted strict rules limiting access to the trail. Permits are required to hike the trail beyond the first 2 miles to Hanakapi'ai Beach, and these are issued on a limited basis.

From the trailhead at Ke'e Beach, climb about 500 feet for the first spectacular views of the Na Pali Coast. The trail then descends to a small ribbon of sand at Hanakapi'ai Beach. From this point on the path becomes much more strenuous. The trail first switchbacks steeply 800 feet above Hanakapi'ai Beach. The trail ahead continues, sometimes skirting towering cliffs hundreds of feet below the trail and sometimes diverting inland to traverse deep jungled valleys.

Hanakoa Valley marks the end of the day-use permit, and a few shaded picnic tables there provide a welcome relief from the heat and demanding trail. An unmaintained 0.4-mile trail up the east fork of the valley to Hanakoa Falls has hazardous, eroded sections, but affords a spectacular view of the falls. From Hanakoa, return to the trailhead at Ke'e Beach by retracing the outward journey in reverse.

WEATHER AND WILDLIFE

Temperatures on the Na Pali Coast seldom drop below 60°F, but summer trade winds bring frequent showers. Be prepared for both soaking rain and stifling midday heat. The trail has little cover, so be wary of sunburn and heat exhaustion. Winter weather is cooler, but less predictable. Be sure to carry plenty of water. It is possible to contract leptospirosis—a potentially fatal disease often mistaken for hepatitis—by drinking untreated stream water. Stream crossings can quickly become dangerous muddy torrents during heavy rainfall. In that case, wait; water levels will recede as quickly as they rose. Also, do not plan to swim. The narrow beaches of the Na Pali Coast are notoriously treacherous, even during summer, and there are no lifeguards or emergency services.

Few animals will be encountered along Kalalau Trail except for feral goats, which are hunted in August and September. Spiders, scorpions, centipedes, and other harmful insects may be found under leaf litter and rocks.

Kalalau Trail and Na Pali Coast

LODGING AND CAMPING

There is no camping at or near the trailhead. If you choose to stay overnight on the trail, backcountry campsites are available at Hanalapi'ai Beach, Hanakoa Valley, and Kalalau Beach. A maximum stay of five nights is allowed along the Kalalau Trail, with no two consecutive nights permitted at Hanakapi'ai or Hanakoa. Campsites at Kalalau Valley are booked nearly a year in advance.

There are no services or lodging at the trailhead in Ha'ena State Park, but both are available 16 miles east in Kilauea.

FEES AND CONTACTS

There are no fees for Ha'ena State Park or for hiking Kalalau Trail.

Permits for hiking or camping on the trail are free and may be requested in person or by mail at Kauai State Parks Office, 3060 Eiwa Street, Room 306, Lihu'e, HI 96766, or by phone at (808) 274-3445. Day-use permits are granted no farther than Hanakoa Valley, about 6.5 miles from the trailhead, and this is where the day hiker should turn back. More information can be found at the Kauai State Park Web site, **www.hawaiistateparks.org/parks/kauai.**

14 CHILKOOT TRAIL

Location: *Klondike Gold Rush National Historic Park, Skagway, AK*
Distance: *16.4 miles*
Elevation Extremes: *65 feet to 600 feet*
Total Elevation Gain: *1,700 feet*
Difficulty: *Very Strenuous*
USGS Maps: *Skagway C-1 22.5-minute*
Trailhead Coordinates: *N 59° 30' 41.9" W 135° 20' 48.0"*
UTM 8V 0480370 6597060 [WGS 84]

THE GOLDEN STAIRS

Newspaper headlines in 1897 read "GOLD!!" and thousands of Americans, worn down by economic depression, sold their farms and businesses and boarded ships to follow their dreams north. Most disembarked at Skagway—the northern outpost of Alaska's Inside Passage waterway—and followed Chilkoot Trail from the coast to the Yukon gold fields. Their unprecedented display of hope, determination, and physical endurance lives on in a faded but famous black-and-white photo. It captured the treasure-seekers trudging up a snowy pass known as "the golden stairs." A few, perhaps some in that very photo, struck gold. Many more returned home penniless but richer for the adventure. Modern hikers come away with the same exhalted feeling.

I still remember the first time I saw a picture of "the golden stairs." Hundreds of prospectors were trudging up a snowy pass in a faded black-and-white photo. It was an unprecedented display of hope, determination, and physical endurance.

A direct flight to Skagway was too expensive, so I settled for landing in Juneau, the capital of Alaska, and took an overnight ferry that delivered me to Skagway at 5:30 a.m. It was late September, so Alaska's famed arc of summertime daylight would be down to about 13 hours now. I had no time to waste getting on the trail.

I had no idea how to get from the ferry terminal to the trailhead in Dyea, so I asked the attendant at the ferry ticket window. After an early morning call to Dyea Dave, a taxi driver, Ruth McClelland, picked me up in a minivan and drove me up rough roads along the Taiya River for nearly 30 minutes. Ruth was a wealth of information. She told me that the native Tinglit called this area the "valley of the screaming

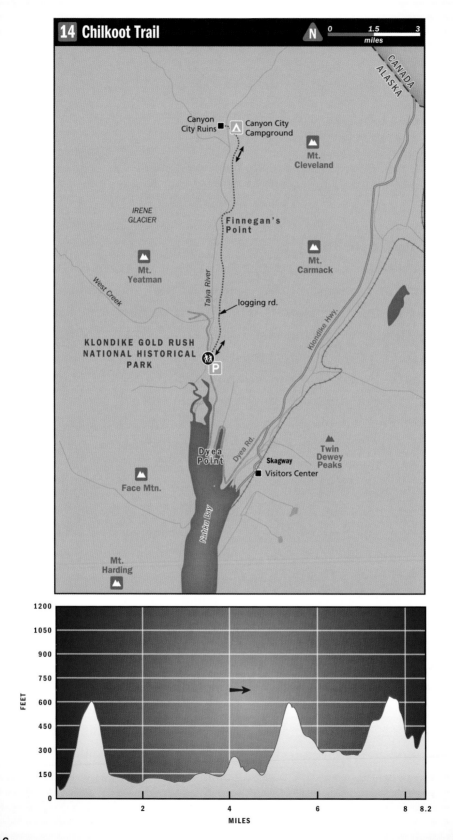

wind." She also warned me to ". . . watch out for bears and make plenty of noise. There have been a lot of bear encounters lately, although only one person has been mauled." I think that last part was supposed to make me feel better.

The tide was going out on the Taiya River, and I counted five eagles sitting on the shoals as we neared the trailhead. They were no doubt hoping that the outgoing tide would leave an easy meal or two. Ruth dropped me off on the legendary Chilkoot Trail at 7:15 a.m., and promised to pick me up again at 3 p.m. In that amount of time, I hoped that I would be able to reach the ruins of Canyon City, 8.2 miles from the trailhead, and return. That wouldn't be a problem if the trail was well maintained and relatively flat, but the trail quickly proved to be much more difficult than I had imagined. The first half mile of trail was terrible, gaining about 500 feet over rocky, steep terrain. Unless the character of the trail changed for the better, I would not be able to reach my goal.

Fortunately, the trail descended again and followed an old logging road along the west bank of the Taiya River. A fog hung heavy in the river valley, limiting visibility to only a few feet, and a different concern soon arose. A pile of bear scat was on the trail every few hundred feet, and fresh bear tracks were everywhere. It was easy to see why from the scat. High bush cranberries were in full fruit, and the bears had all come down for an easy meal. I was the only hiker on the trail, so I nervously broke into an old hiking song:

> *I love to go a-wandering along the mountain track,*
> *and as I go I love to sing, my knapsack on my back.*
> *Valderie, valderah, valderie, valderah,*
> *. . . my knapsack on my back.*

The trail next cut across an extensive series of beaver dams, and the trail crews had built elevated boardwalks through the beaver ponds. Sometimes the boards were two or three inches below water level, and it looked like an amusing competition between the beaver and the trail crews. The beaver would build their dams higher, then the trail crews would raise the boardwalks, then the beaver would build their dams higher, and so on.

I reached Finnegan's Point at 9:05 a.m. Finnegan's Point was named for Pat Finnegan, a man who tried to collect ferry tolls from stampeders. This was as far as wagons could come in summer, although in winter the stampeders could drag their sledges farther up the frozen river. This is also the first campground along the trail, and a tent cabin was set up for campers. A few trails ran uphill from Finnegan's Point, but I finally found Chilkoot Trail continuing upstream along the west bank of the Taiya River.

The trail gained elevation twice to avoid high river cliffs, and then crossed a stream on a bridge that had been moved even farther up the hill. After the bridge, the trail stayed mainly on bottomland, except for one more steep climb and descent before I reached Canyon City camp-site at mile 7.5. Here again, a tent cabin was set up for campers, as well as a log building and a couple of picnic tables. The tables looked inviting, but my schedule required that I press on.

Just before Canyon City the fog parted as if by magic, revealing a breathtaking view of a snow-covered peak far ahead. I wanted desper-ately to see the pass itself, "the golden stairs," where so many stam-peders risked everything for their dreams, but it was still more than

A distant mountain near Canyon City

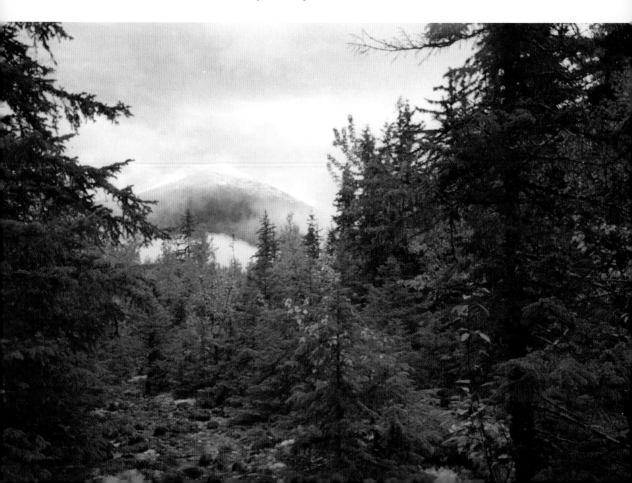

8 miles ahead and hidden from my view. The Canadian North West
Mounted Police wisely required that every prospector carry one ton of
gear and supplies to enter the Yukon, and scales at the pass guaranteed
compliance. Without that regulation, many prospectors simply would
not have survived the arduous terrain and demanding weather. The
fabled "ton of gear" required multiple trips over demanding terrain, fer-
rying the gear from campsite to campsite.

I crossed a swinging bridge at mile 8.0 and entered the ruins of
Canyon City at 10:40 a.m. Nature had done an admirable job of re-
claiming the city, but I could still see several foundations, an old res-
taurant stove, and a large boiler. Because of all the relics along its
length, the Chilkoot Trail is considered the world's longest outdoor
museum. I wanted to continue toward the pass, but this was the place
for me to turn back. It was my goal that a reasonably fit hiker could
accomplish every hike in this book in a single day. A journey to the
Chilkoot Pass and back would be a trek of 31 miles, and although it has
been done in a single day, that would far exceed my objective as well as
my abilities. Canyon City would be far enough this day. I headed back
toward Finnegan's Point and the trailhead.

I arrived back at Finnegan's Point for a late lunch at 12:15 p.m.,
but it looked like a completely different setting. The fog had lifted
revealing glorious snow-covered mountains. High across the river a
craggy glacier spilled from a hanging valley. These are the same spectacular scenes that greeted the stampeders in 1898, and certainly must
have given them pause about the rugged journey ahead.

Back on the trail along the old logging roads, I again saw frequent
bear scat and tracks:

> *I wave my hat to all I see, and they wave back to me,*
> *the blackbird sings so clear and sweet from every greenwood tree.*
> *Valderie, valderah, valderie, valderah,*
> *. . . from every greenwood tree.*

Farther down the trail I saw bear tracks so fresh that the water
was still draining into the depression. Even louder:

> *Oh may I go a-wandering until the day I die,*
> *and may I always laugh and sing beneath God's clear blue sky.*
> *Valderie, valderah, valderie, valderah,*
> *. . . beneath God's clear blue sky.*

When I finally reached the trailhead at 2:30 p.m., I was not only tired from the difficult hike, but hoarse from singing so loudly. I was back early so I took out my cell phone, was pleased to see I was in range, and made a call to Dyea Dave for an early pickup. In a few minutes my taxi appeared and I was headed back to Skagway. The tide was in during the drive back down the Taiya River, and sea otters were playing in the shallows, replacing the eagles I saw earlier. After stopping for a few minutes at the Klondike Gold Rush National Historic Park Visitor Center in Skagway, I caught the ferry back to Juneau at 4:30 p.m.

The ferry ride back down the inside passage to Juneau, this time accomplished in the daylight, was pure magic. The sunset bathed spectacular snow-covered peaks in a rosy glow, while humpback whales played in the still waters off the ferry bow. It was a fitting conclusion to an extremely memorable day.

Key Trail Points

From the trailhead in Dyea on the Taiya River:
  1.6 miles to the Old Logging Road junction
  4.8 miles to Finnegan's Point
  7.5 miles to the Canyon City campground
  8.2 miles to Canyon City
  16.4 miles to return to the trailhead in Dyea

DIRECTIONS TO TRAILHEAD AND TRAIL ROUTE

Direct flights may be taken to Skagway or Whitehorse, Yukon, but these flights are typically expensive. It is less costly to fly to Juneau and book a ferry to Skagway. From Skagway a taxi or shuttle must be arranged to carry you 8.5 miles on the Dyea Road to the trailhead. The trailhead is located just before Dyea Road crosses Taiya River.

Chilkoot Trail leads north from the trailhead, sometimes on level ground and sometimes climbing sharply to skirt river cliffs. Take the trail north to Finnegan's Point, Canyon City, and return. There are no other trails or trail junctions to cause confusion.

WEATHER AND WILDLIFE

The climate on Chilkoot Trail is basically a maritime climate with cool summers and mild winters. Average daily highs in summer are 59° to 67°F, while average winter lows are 16° to 27°F. Summer days range from cool and rainy to warm and sunny. Skagway, averaging only 26 inches of rainfall per year, is drier than the rainforest climate farther south, where the coast from Juneau to Ketchikan averages 90 to 160 inches of rain per year. September and October are the rainiest months on the Chilkoot.

Wildlife commonly seen along the Chilkoot Trail includes bald eagles, sea otters, beavers, and bears.

LODGING AND CAMPING

There is no lodging in Dyea. Services in Skagway include the Westmark Inn, a reasonably priced hotel, as well as a few bed-and-breakfasts.

Dyea Campground is open daily when free of snow. There are 22 sites for vehicle or walk-in camping; the fee is $10 per night. Campgrounds along Chilkoot Trail require a backcountry permit from June 1 to September 5. A permit for camping on the U.S. side of the trail is about $18, and for the entire trail about $50. Backcountry permits can be reserved in advance for an additional fee; call (800) 661-0486.

FEES AND CONTACTS

There is no fee for parking or day use of Chilkoot Trail. Multiday permits are required, as listed above.

The ferry to Skagway can be booked with the Alaska Marine Highway Ferry System, Reservations, PO Box 112505, Juneau, AK 99811-2505, or by phone at (907) 465-3941. Information regarding fares and schedules can be obtained at their Web site at **www.dot.state.ak.us/amhs.** The round-trip fare was $100 for my trip, but fares vary seasonally. For questions regarding conditions and use of the Chilkoot Trail, contact Klondike Gold Rush National Historic Park, PO Box 517, Skagway, AK 99840, or by phone at (907) 983-2921. The park Web site is **www.nps.gov/klgo.**

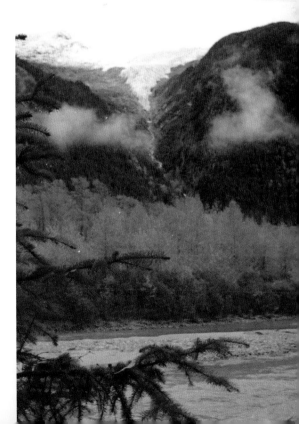

Taiya River and Irene Glacier from Finnegan's Point

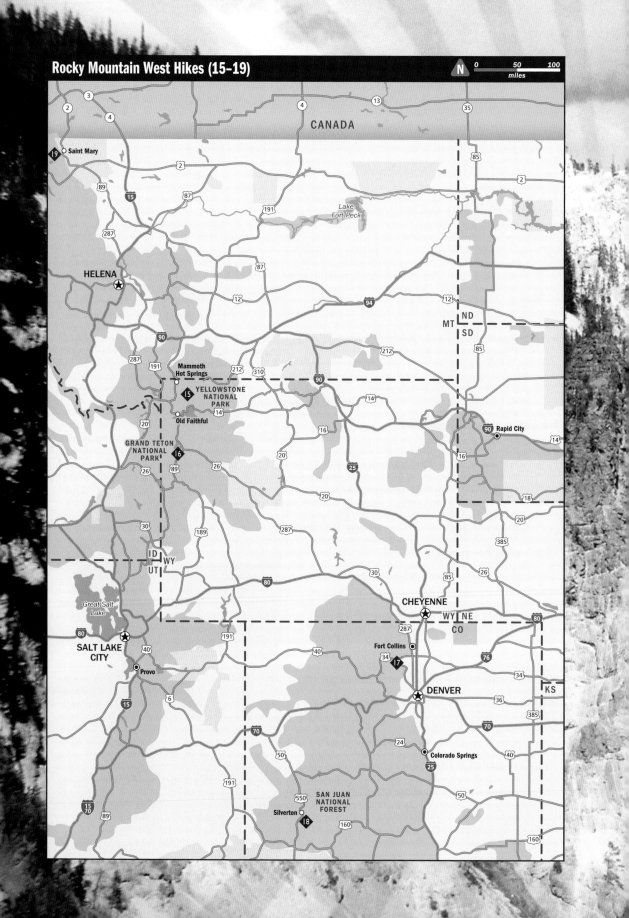

Rocky Mountain West Hikes (15–19)

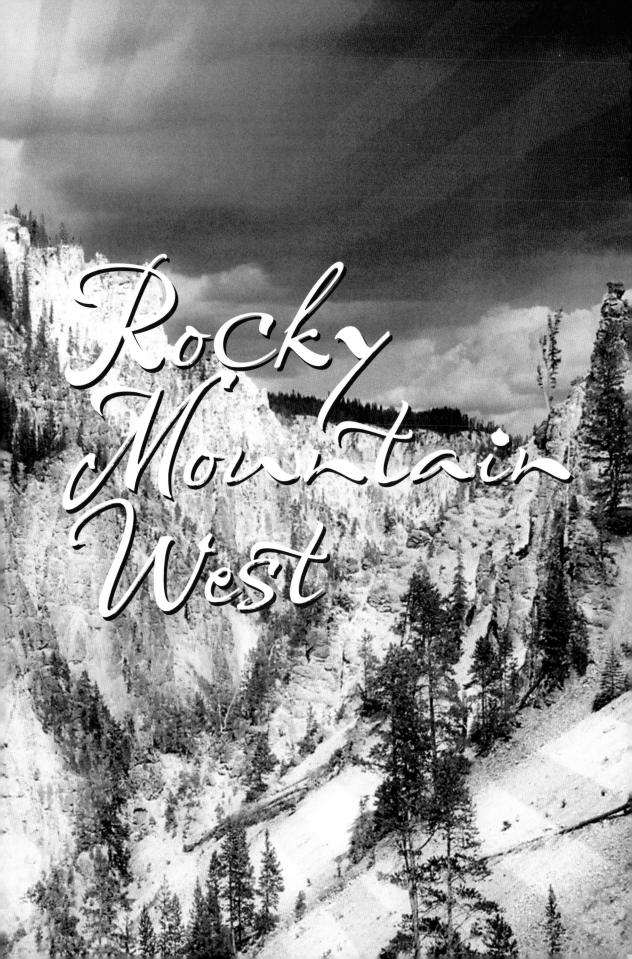

Rocky Mountain West

15 GRAND CANYON OF THE YELLOWSTONE LOOP
(CLEAR LAKE, RIBBON LAKE, AND SOUTH RIM TRAILS)

Location: *Yellowstone National Park, WY*
Distance: *4.9 miles*
Elevation Extremes: *7,200 to 7,940 feet*
Total Elevation Gain: *910 feet*
Difficulty: *Moderate*
USGS Maps: *Canyon Village 7.5-minute*
Trailhead Coordinates: *N 44° 42' 49.0" W 110° 29' 46.4"*
                               UTM 12T 0540044 4951265 [WGS 84]

A NATIONAL TREASURE

Yellowstone wears a unique mantle as the first national park in the world. President Ulysses S. Grant presented an enduring gift to the American people when he signed legislation in 1872 to establish protective boundaries around this natural wonderland. Since then, more than 50 other U.S. national parks have been created, yet Yellowstone remains unique. What other park can boast such an assortment of geysers and hot springs that its total exceeds the combined number of those found on the rest of the planet? In addition, Yellowstone has a waterfall twice as high as Niagara Falls and a canyon so deep and beautiful that it can only be called grand. Add to these features an assortment of Rocky Mountain animals collectively found only in Yellowstone National Park.

Although Yellowstone is widely known for its thermal features, this hike focuses on one of America's great national treasures, the Grand Canyon of the Yellowstone. True, the scale of this canyon is smaller than that of the Grand Canyon in Arizona, but many consider the Grand Canyon of the Yellowstone to be more distinctive and beautiful than its southwestern counterpart. In addition to the Grand Canyon of the Yellowstone, this hike also includes seldom-visited thermal features, backwoods lakes, and a distant view of Hayden Valley.

My family and I had just driven through Hayden Valley on our way from Old Faithful to Canyon; we were astonished at the abundance of wildlife there. It was early August, and the valley was literally black with bison that rolled across the grassland and flowed like a

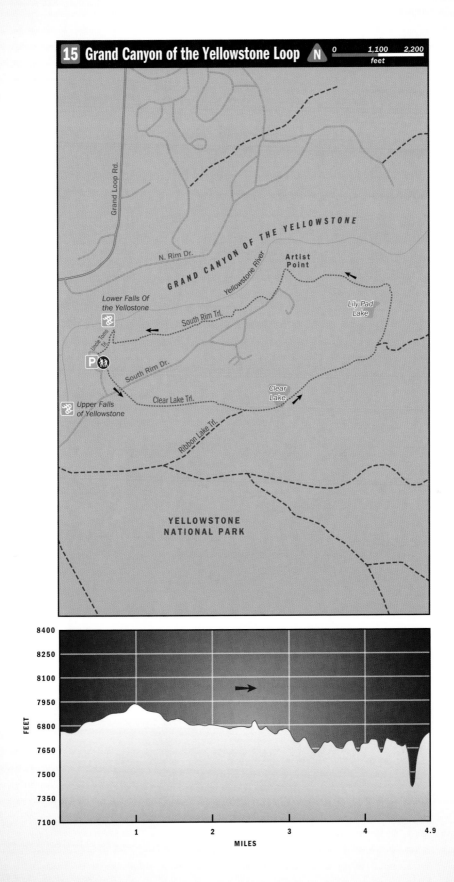

15 Grand Canyon of the Yellowstone Loop

N

0   1,100   2,200
feet

Grand Loop Rd.

N. Rim Dr.

GRAND CANYON OF THE YELLOWSTONE

Yellowstone River

Artist Point

Lower Falls Of the Yellostone

South Rim Trl.

Lily Pad Lake

Uncle Toms Trl.

P

South Rim Dr.

Clear Lake Trl.

Clear Lake

Upper Falls of Yellowstone

Ribbon Lake Trl.

YELLOWSTONE NATIONAL PARK

FEET

8400
8250
8100
7950
6800
7650
7500
7350
7100

1   2   3   4   4.9

MILES

relentless tide around the stopped cars. I expected our Grand Canyon of the Yellowstone hike to be impressive, but Hayden Valley would be a tough act to follow.

We parked in Uncle Tom's Parking Area, crossed South Rim Drive, and started up Clear Lake Trail by early afternoon. We first came to a sign warning "bear country," and advising not to hike alone and to check with rangers for local bear conditions—good advice. Soon we came to a junction with Ribbon Lake Trail, and I couldn't resist walking off-trail to the top of an open ridge for a view toward the south. The ridge gave a distant vista all the way to the eastern part of Hayden Valley, but there was no sign of the bison herds that had impressed us only three hours earlier. We turned left onto Ribbon Lake Trail toward Clear Lake.

The trail to Clear Lake was gentle and shady, and we soon arrived at the lake, but it was not what I had imagined from its name. It was a thermal body, filled with mineral water and the white skeletons of long-dead trees. What really drew our attention was to the right: Rising

Lilypad Lake

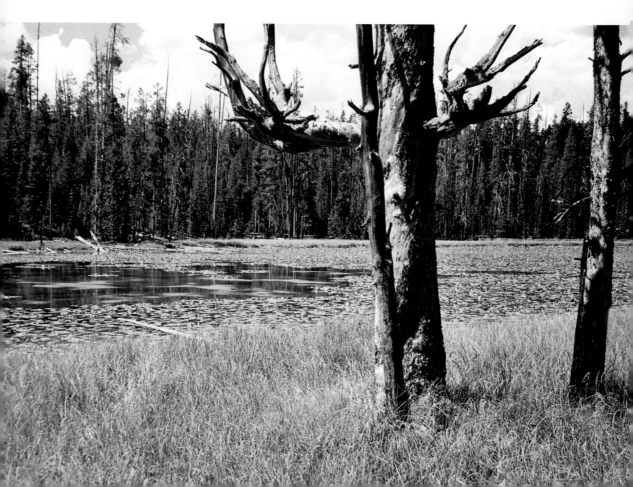

steam turned out to be a small collection of mud pots burping comically into the air. The distinctive quality of the mud pots, the hissing of the steam vents, and the pungent smell of sulfur took on a special quality here in the backwoods away from the tourists that throng the major attractions of the park. Back on the trail, we soon passed other steam vents and fumaroles before coming to another trail junction. Here we turned left away from the thermal activity and into a heavy lodgepole-pine forest.

Soon after the trail junction we came to Lily Pad Lake, and the contrast with Clear Lake could not have been greater. True to its name, Lily Pad Lake was crammed with lily pads and other plants and was bordered by lush lodgepole-pine forest. We continued over a rise of land, suddenly emerged from the forest, and there it was!

It is difficult to put into words the first impact of the Grand Canyon of the Yellowstone. Delicate hues of yellow, orange, and red painted the canyon walls in an ever-changing panorama of light and mood. Puffs of steam betrayed hydrothermal activity in the canyon walls that remind us of its dynamic geologic history. The scene was stunning, and made even more so by the fact that this place was not readily accessible. Here we saw the canyon as it once was, without asphalt paving and steel fences, and without the crowds of tourists elbowing each other for a place at the rail. As Nathaniel Langford, one of the first explorers to record his impressions of the Grand Canyon of the Yellowstone said, "As I took in the scene, I realized my own littleness, my helplessness, my dread exposure to destruction, my inability to cope with or even comprehend the mighty architecture of nature. . . ."

We continued west along the trail a short distance to the infamous Artist Point. Artist Point is regarded as the most beautiful of the many vistas on the rim of the canyon, and it was easy to understand why. Here the magnificent Lower Falls of the Yellowstone came into full view. At the head of the canyon, Yellowstone River dropped over a resistant ledge of rhyolite lava to plunge 308 feet and carve the canyon 1,000 feet deep.

From Artist Point we quickly walked to the west end of the parking area and found South Rim Trail. South Rim Trail continued generally west but frequently dropped away from the canyon when it encountered a small valley, then climbed back to the rim for another jaw-dropping viewpoint on the opposite side.

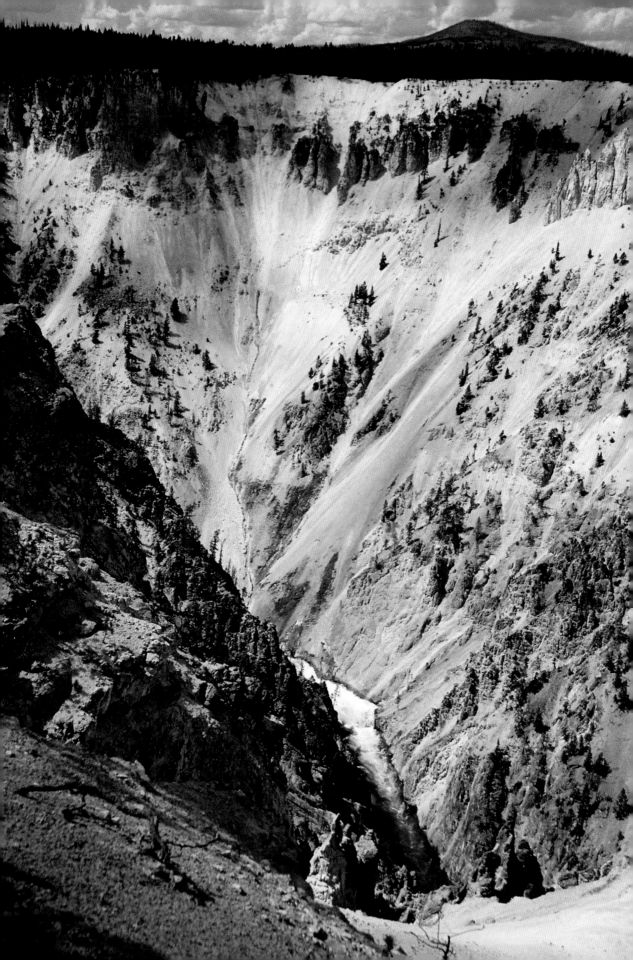

We reached the junction with Uncle Tom's Trail, which descended 500 feet to the bottom. The trail, in fact, is named for "Uncle" Tom Richardson, who in the early 1900s led visitors down 528 steps and rope ladders to the river, rowed them across the torrent, and took them up to the North Rim.

As I descended the trail—alone now—the power of the cascade became more palpable, and at the final platform the Lower Falls thundered its presence. As much as 63,000 gallons of water plunge over the brink of the falls every second to carve the canyon ever deeper. A brilliant rainbow played in the mist, and the walls of the canyon were lush green from the constant spray. I knew that the climb back up the steep trail would be tough, but being in this unique place was easily worth the effort.

I returned to the South Rim Trail and to Uncle Tom's Trail parking area where my family was waiting. We took a short walk to view the Upper Falls before heading off in hopes of observing gray wolves in Lamar Valley. The beauty of the Grand Canyon of the Yellowstone, the power of the Lower Falls, as well as the quiet appeal of the lodgepole-pine forest and seldom-visited thermal activity, make this one of the most memorable short loop trails I had ever experienced.

Key Trail Points

From the trailhead at Uncle Tom's Trail parking area:
- 1.2 miles to Clear Lake
- 2.0 miles to Lily Pad Lake
- 2.7 miles to Artist Point
- 4.5 miles to Uncle Tom's Trail
- 4.9 miles to trailhead at Uncle Tom's Trail parking area

DIRECTIONS TO TRAILHEAD AND TRAIL ROUTE

To reach the trailhead from Canyon Village Junction, travel 2.4 miles south on the main road toward Yellowstone Lake, then turn left onto South Rim Drive. Cross Chittenden Bridge over the river, and after 0.5 miles turn left into Uncle Tom's Trail parking area.

From the trailhead at the parking area, cross South Rim Drive and

Canyon of the Yellowstone

hike 1.2 miles on Clear Lake Trail to Clear Lake. Pass Clear Lake and continue onto Ribbon Lake Trail past interesting mud pots and thermal vents to a trail junction just south of Lily Pad Lake. Turn north past Lily Pad Lake and climb over a height of land to suddenly overlook the Grand Canyon of the Yellowstone. The impact of emerging from the trees to such grandeur is unforgettable.

Walk west along the South Rim to Artist Point, 0.7 miles west of Lily Pad Lake. From Artist Point, walk to the west end of the Artist Point parking lot and locate the South Rim Trailhead. Follow the South Rim Trail back to the Uncle Tom's Trail parking area. But just before returning to your car, turn north onto Uncle Tom's Trail for a unique canyon experience. Descend 500 feet down steep inclines and 528 steps to a spectacular viewpoint near the base of the Lower Falls. Uncle Tom's Trail may be icy in the early morning, and the trail is subject to closure in spring and fall due to snow and ice. Retrace Uncle Tom's Trail back up to the South Rim, and return to the parking area.

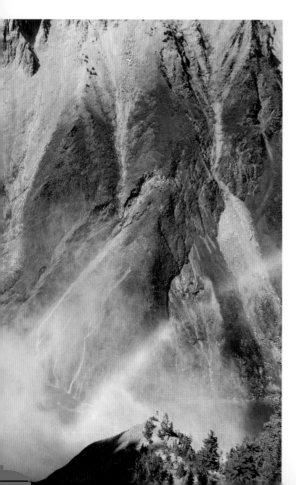

Yellowstone Falls from Uncle Tom's Trail

WEATHER AND WILDLIFE

Summer in Yellowstone is characterized by highs in the 70s and cool nights, although thunderstorms in the afternoon are common. Daytime temperatures in spring and fall can range from the 30s to 60s, and weather can be unpredictable with sudden changes. Snowfalls of up to 12 inches are not uncommon in spring and fall, and roads may be temporarily closed due to heavy snow. Roads to Canyon and Old Faithful typically close about the first of November. Park roads to Old Faithful usually open in late April; roads to the Lake and Canyon areas open in early May.

One of the highlights of Yellowstone is the amazing abundance of Rocky Mountain animals, including wolves, elk, bison, deer, bighorn sheep, grizzly bears, black bears, moose, pronghorn antelope, mountain lions, coyotes, beavers, trumpeter swans, eagles, ospreys, pelicans, and more. Many of them are so common that even the casual visitor driving through the park will glimpse scores of these animals. Hayden Valley, just north of the Grand Canyon of the Yellowstone, is one of the best places to observe them. Lamar Valley is the best place for wolf-watching.

LODGING AND CAMPING

There are nine lodges within Yellowstone Park, some of them among the great classic inns of America. Both Canyon Lodge and Lake Lodge are convenient as home base for hiking in the Grand Canyon of the Yellowstone area. I have enjoyed staying at Lake Lodge, where bison stroll among the rustic cabins. But the most unforgettable place to stay in Yellowtone is Old Faithful Inn, perhaps the grandest of the old National Park Lodges. Granted, the furnishings are rustic, and sometimes the bathrooms are down the hall, but the character and aura of this magnificent lodge cannot be matched anywhere. The Inn is generally open from mid-May until mid-October, and Xanterra Parks & Resorts begins taking reservations December 15 for the following year. The more rustic, historic rooms range from $98 to $125 per night.

Several campgrounds are available throughout the park. Reservations can be made for some campgrounds, and others are available on a first-come, first-serve basis. All campgrounds in the Yellowstone Park fill up early.

FEES AND CONTACTS

The entry fee for Yellowstone Park is $25 per vehicle for a seven-day pass. Lodge and campground reservations must usually be made several months in advance for Yellowstone and can be obtained from Xanterra Parks & Resorts at (307) 344-7311 or online at **www.yellow stonenationalparklodges.com.**

For additional information, including trail, weather, and bear conditions, contact the Superintendent, PO Box 168, Yellowstone National Park, WY 82190, or phone (307) 344-7381. The park's Web site is at **www.nps.gov/yell**.

16 AMPHITHEATER LAKE– TETON GLACIER TRAIL

Location: *Grand Teton National Park, WY*
Distance: *12.6 miles*
Elevation Extremes: *6,750 to 10,950 feet*
Total Elevation Gain: *4,500 feet*
Difficulty: *Very Strenuous*
USGS Maps: *Grand Teton 7.5-minute*
Trailhead Coordinates: *N 43° 44' 4.7" W 110° 44' 29.4"*
UTM 12T 0520817 4842438 [WGS 84]

IN THE HALL OF THE MOUNTAIN KING

America is blessed with many lovely mountain ranges, but the most beautiful and inspiring of all are the central peaks of the Grand Teton Range, especially when viewed from the northern end of Jackson Hole. Here the Cathedral Group of mountains—which includes Grand Teton, Mount Owen, and Teewinot Mountain—soar upward with stunning abruptness to naked granite pinnacles that rise 7,000 feet above the valley floor. This is one of the steepest mountain fronts, and one of the boldest spectacles of natural scenery in America. The grandeur of the scene is vastly enhanced by the flatness of the valley floor and the absence of any foothills.

This hike to the Teton Glacier, if followed in its entirety, is not for the faint of heart. It first follows a well-worn trail to scenic Amphitheater Lake nestled in a cirque at the top of Disappointment Peak, and then continues across a precarious ledge and glacial moraine onto the surface of Teton Glacier. The final 1.5 miles beyond Amphitheater Lake is not an officially maintained trail, but follows a rough track worn by mountain climbers en route to some of the most renown mountain climbs in the world. At the end of the hike, deep in the heart of the Cathedral Group, the hiker finds himself in one of the most magnificent glacial cirques in North America.

I arose early at our motel to tackle this difficult hike. The peaks of the Teton Range were just beginning to glow pink in the predawn light as I drove north to the Lupine Meadows Trailhead. I was on the trail at 6 a.m., a good time to see the local wildlife. I counted 13 deer on the way up to Surprise Lake, including three does with their fawns.

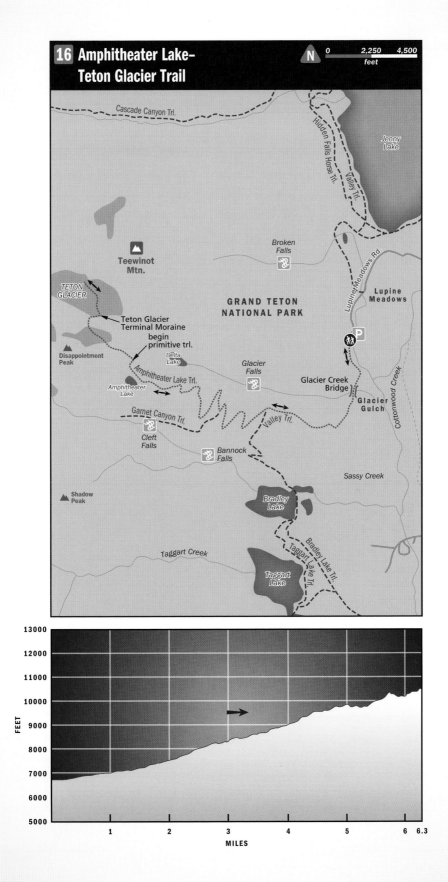

16 Amphitheater Lake–
Teton Glacier Trail

N

0   2,250   4,500
feet

Cascade Canyon Trl.

Hidden Falls Horse Trl.

Valley Trl.

Jenny
Lake

Teewinot
Mtn.

Broken
Falls

TETON
GLACIER

GRAND TETON
NATIONAL PARK

Lupine Meadows Rd.

Lupine
Meadows

Teton Glacier
Terminal Moraine
begin
primitive trl.

Disappointment
Peak

Delta
Lake

Glacier
Falls

P

Amphitheater Lake Trl.

Amphitheater
Lake

Glacier Creek
Bridge

Glacier
Gulch

Cottonwood Creek

Garnet Canyon Trl.

Valley Trl.

Cleft
Falls

Bannock
Falls

Sassy Creek

Shadow
Peak

Bradley
Lake

Taggart Creek

Bradley Lake Trl.

Taggart Lake Trl.

Taggart
Lake

FEET

13000
12000
11000
10000
9000
8000
7000
6000
5000

1   2   3   4   5   6 6.3

MILES

Marmot and Rocky Mountain grouse were also plentiful along the trail that morning. As I climbed higher, the sun warmed the slopes, and the familiar aroma of sage and grasses filled the air. The golden valley of Jackson Hole, that famous rendezvous of the mountain men, unfolded at my feet. I reached Surprise Lake at 8:45 a.m. and arrived at Amphitheater Lake 15 minutes later. I continued on to the notch above Amphitheater Lake and took a snack break with an awe-inspiring vista into Glacier Gulch below.

The steel cable long used as a handhold for the traverse below Disappointment Peak had been removed, so I descended the steep trail east of the ledge and then crossed west under the cliffs of the peak. After traversing the ledge, I struggled up the snow gully and on to the top of the first moraine. Here I paused to absorb what lay before me: The east ridge of the Grand Teton dominated the scene to the west. The great cliffs of the north face of Disappointment Peak, so named because climbers once hoped its gentle slopes would provide an easy route to the summit of the Grand Teton, soared above me on the south. Between the two mountains, an improbable array of jagged pinnacles—the Red Sentinel, Fair Share

Cathedral Group of the Tetons from Jackson Hole

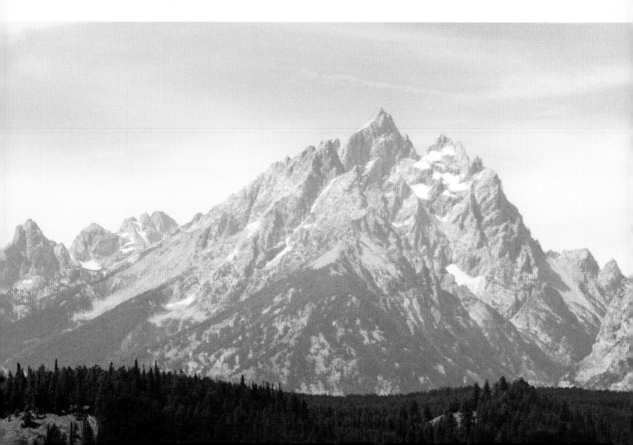

Tower, Pemmican Pinnacle, and Teepe Pillar—pierced the skyline.

I scrambled across seemingly endless boulders and climbed the huge terminal moraine guarding the Teton Glacier. Once on the moraine, I was shocked to see how much the glacier had receded since I first climbed here in 1967. Getting down to the toe of the glacier now required a delicate traverse across loose scree. It was all more difficult than I remembered.

Finally on the glacier itself, I crossed small crevasses and meltwater channels, and hiked to the rock walls beneath Mount Owen by late morning. Fearsome cliffs towered on all sides of me. Teewinot Mountain, named for a Shoshone word meaning "pinnacles," rose to the east, silhouetted against the brown and gold of Jackson Hole. Mount Owen, the most difficult peak in the Teton Range to climb, towered behind me. Dominating the scene to the south was the infamous North Face of the Grand Teton. From this vantage point, the North Face looked complex and threatening. First climbed in its entirety in 1949, this face remained one of the great mountaineering routes in North America for decades. As a young man of 23, I headed up that face together with Greg Joiner, my teenage climbing partner. Truth is, we were in over our heads, but two days later we completed the route and finally stood on the summit. One of my most enduring memories was leading the notorious pendulum pitch, a hand traverse with nothing for the feet, hanging 2,000 feet above the Teton Glacier. It all seemed a very long time ago.

After reminiscing awhile, I turned my back on this amazing place and headed down, across the crevasses and meltwater channels of the glacier, across the two terminal moraines, and back up the ledge beneath the cliffs of Disappointment Peak. I paused for a late lunch at the notch above Amphitheater Lake before finally heading down the trail toward Lupine Meadows. The trail was still congested with day-hikers struggling to reach Amphitheater Lake and asking how far it was at every switchback. I reached Lupine Meadows and the parking lot at about 3 p.m., completing a nine-hour trek.

This very rugged but spectacular route is without a doubt one of the best mountain hikes in America. The craggy spires and intimidating rock walls of the Cathedral Group leave a lasting impression of the exciting and perilous world of the serious mountaineer. Even those who decide to turn back at the notch above Amphitheater Lake have still completed one of the country's best hikes.

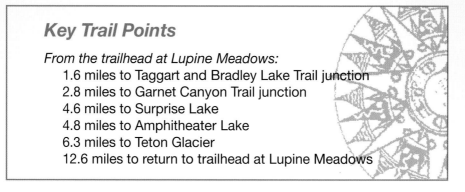

Key Trail Points

From the trailhead at Lupine Meadows:
    1.6 miles to Taggart and Bradley Lake Trail junction
    2.8 miles to Garnet Canyon Trail junction
    4.6 miles to Surprise Lake
    4.8 miles to Amphitheater Lake
    6.3 miles to Teton Glacier
    12.6 miles to return to trailhead at Lupine Meadows

DIRECTIONS TO TRAILHEAD AND TRAIL ROUTE

To reach the trailhead, drive 6.6 miles north of the Moose Entrance Station on Teton Park Road. Turn left at Lupine Meadows Junction and follow signs to the Lupine Meadows Trailhead. If coming south from Jenny Lake, Lupine Meadows Junction is less than a mile from South Jenny Lake. From the trailhead, follow Glacier Trail past junctions that lead to Taggart Lake and Garnet Canyon to Surprise Lake, which is 2,800 feet and 19 switchbacks above Lupine Meadows. Just beyond Surprise Lake is beautiful Amphitheater Lake at an elevation of about 9,700 feet. For most day-hikers, this is the goal and a place to turn back.

From Amphitheater Lake, follow unmaintained trails leading right to a notch on the north skyline for a breathtaking view down into Glacier Gulch. From this point on, memorize the route well for the return journey later in the day. Follow the track down the far (north) side for about 150 feet until it angles left on a ledge under the sheer north cliffs of Disappointment Peak. Steel cables anchored to the rock once protected hikers on the exposed eastern end of this ledge, but the cables have long since been removed. Without the cable as a handhold, it may be more comfortable to descend the steep trail east of the ledge, and then traverse west to the base of the most exposed section. Traverse the ledge west beneath the north cliffs of Disappointment Peak, aiming for the snow-filled gully ahead. Early in the season, steep and dangerous snow slopes will cover the ledge. This traverse should not be attempted before late July without an ice ax and crampons and the skill to use them.

Once in the gully, ascend the snow until the angle becomes uncomfortable, and then climb right, up boulders

Grand Teton at sunrise on
Amphitheater Lake Trail

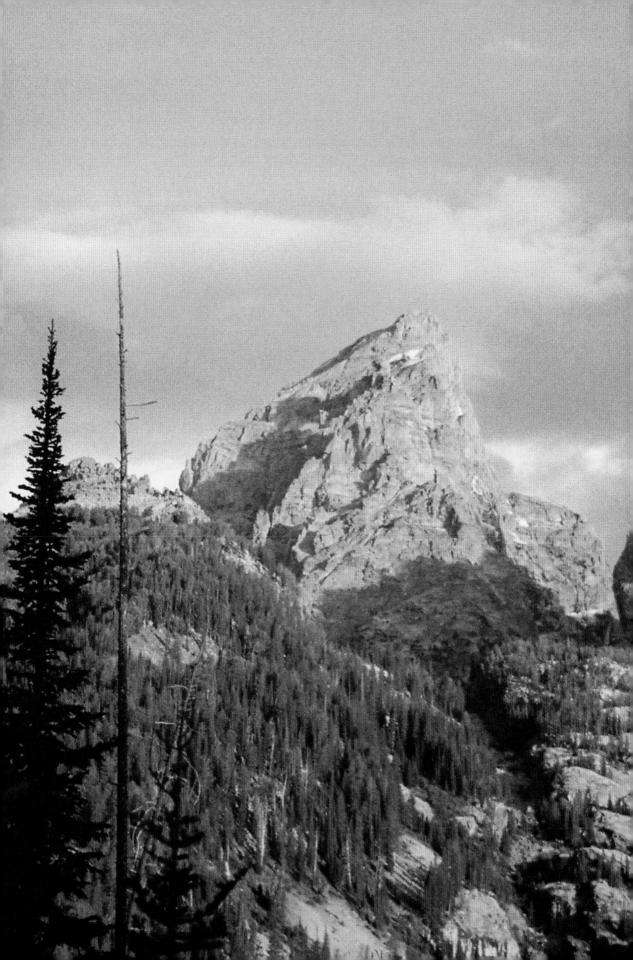

and scree, to the top of the first glacier moraine. There is no trail here. Descend the far side of the moraine, and then cross boulders to the Teton Glacier terminal moraine. This moraine is best ascended at its left (west) edge against the east ridge of the Grand Teton. In the 1920s it was possible to step a few feet down from the crest of the moraine onto the surface of the glacier, but now it is necessary to follow the moraine east for 200 to 300 feet and then negotiate a tricky steep traverse back to the left. Next, climb the rubble slope above, which is actually the rock-strewn surface of Teton Glacier. Crest the front of the glacier and cross small crevasses and meltwater channels to the great cliffs directly beneath Mount Owen. Do not climb farther onto the upper level of the Teton Glacier due to danger from falling rock.

This is not an easy place to reach. The last 1.5 miles is especially rugged and demanding. But for those who persevere, the reward is a rare glimpse into the heady world of the mountain climber. Two of the 50 great classic climbs of America loom directly overhead: the North Face and North Ridge of the Grand Teton. Seemingly impossible rock walls, threatening yet exciting, soar on almost every side. Return by retracing the route across the glacial moraines and past Amphitheater Lake back to the Lupine Meadows Trailhead.

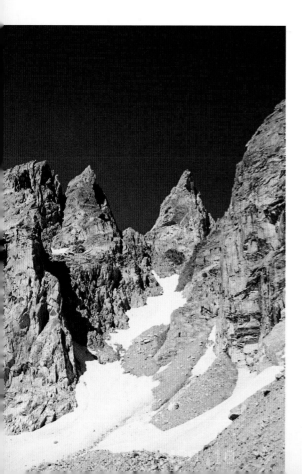

Pinnacles and spires from the Teton Glacier

It is no longer necessary to register off-trail scrambling with the park rangers, but be sure to let someone know your destination and schedule before attempting this difficult hike.

WEATHER AND WILDLIFE
Spring in Jackson Hole is characterized by mild days and cool nights. The valley is generally covered with snow until late May, and parts of the trail to Teton Glacier will likely be covered with

snow until late July. From late July to early September, mornings are usually clear, with afternoon thunderstorms not uncommon. Some of these thunderstorms can be quite severe. These storms almost always come from the southwest, which means there is very little warning for hikers on the eastern side of the range. The highest percentage of clear days occurs in August, and the first winter storm does not ordinarily hit until the end of the first week of September.

Most of the animals common in Yellowstone are also present in Grand Teton National Park. Moose, elk, mule deer, bison, and prong-horn antelope are common. Grizzly bears, black bears, and mountain lions are more elusive. Pikas, yellow-bellied marmots, and ground squirrels are common in the high country.

LODGING AND CAMPING

There are several options for lodging both in and outside the park. Most convenient for this hike are the Coulter Bay Cabins, Jackson Lake Lodge, and Jenny Lake Lodge. There is also an American Alpine Club Climbers Ranch near Jenny Lake. Several other options for lodging and services can be found in or near Jackson, Wyoming.

There are more than 900 campsites available in five full-service campgrounds in the park. The largest are Coulter Bay Campground on Jackson Lake and Gros Ventre Campground in the north end of the park. These campgrounds rarely fill up. Jenny Lake Campground, with 51 sites for tents only, is more coveted and usually fills by 11 a.m. For those who wish to split this demanding hike into two days, there are a limited number of backcountry campsites at Amphitheater Lake. These can be reserved at the Ranger Station at Jenny Lake. Reservations for lodges and campgrounds inside the park can be made online at **www.gtlc.com,** or by calling (800) 628-9988.

FEES AND CONTACTS

The entrance fee for Grand Teton National Park is $25 per day per vehicle for seven days, and the same pass can be used for entry into Yellowstone Park.

For more information, write the Superintendent, Grand Teton National Park, PO Drawer 170, Moose, WY 83012-0170, or phone (307) 739-3300. The park Web site is **www.nps.gov/grte.**

17 **LONGS PEAK TRAIL**

Location: *Rocky Mountain National Park, CO*
Distance: *15 miles*
Elevation Extremes: *9,400 to 14,255 feet*
Total Elevation Gain: *4,900 feet*
Difficulty: *Very Strenuous*
USGS Map: *Longs Peak 7.5-minute*
Trailhead Coordinates: *N 40° 16' 21.0" W 110° 44' 29.4"*
UTM 13T 0452626 4458150 [WGS 84]

ROCKY MOUNTAIN RITE OF PASSAGE

Longs Peak in Rocky Mountain National Park has every quality that makes a mountain memorable. It is the northernmost 14,000-foot peak in the Rockies, and one of three landmark high points of the Front Range. The Keyhole Route, the only nontechnical hike to the summit of Longs Peak, has traditionally been considered a rite of passage for serious hikers in Colorado and surrounding states. In fact, Longs Peak is the most-climbed high peak in America, with about 10,000 people striving for its summit each year. If you are looking for solitude and a true wilderness experience, look elsewhere. But if what you crave is a challenging scramble over spectacular precipitous terrain in the company of many other pilgrims, all striving for the same lofty goal, then this famous hike is not to be missed.

John Wesley Powell first climbed Longs Peak in 1868 after other members of his party declared it "unclimbable." The one-armed Powell forced his way along the Traverse and Homestretch, the upper portion of what is now known as the Keyhole Route, and onto the summit plateau. It was an achievement that first brought acclaim to the pioneer who would later become the first explorer to descend the Colorado River through the Grand Canyon.

I pulled into the parking lot at Longs Peak Ranger Station in the dark at 2:30 a.m. and was shocked to see it already packed. Not only that, but the shoulder of the road also was full of vehicles for 200 yards toward CO 7 as well. Not wanting to add elevation to my hike, I drove over toward Longs Peak Campground and found a good spot along the road. I filled my water bottles at the campground, switched on my headlamp, and started up the trail toward Longs Peak at 2:45 a.m.

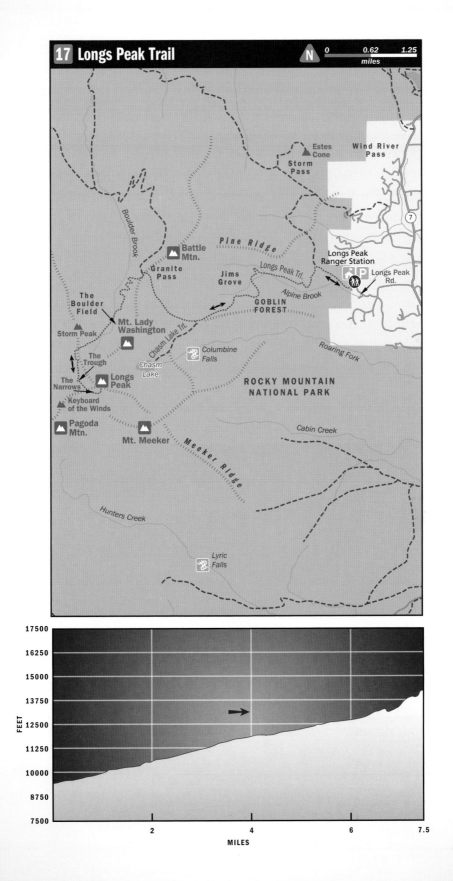

17 Longs Peak Trail

N

0   0.62   1.25
miles

Estes Cone

Wind River Pass

Storm Pass

Boulder Brook

Pine Ridge

Battle Mtn.

Granite Pass

Jims Grove

Longs Peak Trl.

Longs Peak Ranger Station

The Boulder Field

Alpine Brook

Longs Peak Rd.

Storm Peak

Mt. Lady Washington

GOBLIN FOREST

The Trough

Chasm Lake Trl.

Columbine Falls

The Narrows

Chasm Lake

Roaring Fork

Longs Peak

ROCKY MOUNTAIN NATIONAL PARK

Keyboard of the Winds

Pagoda Mtn.

Mt. Meeker

Meeker Ridge

Cabin Creek

Hunters Creek

Lyric Falls

Several other hikers were on the trail that morning, all shining little pools of light in the darkness. Once above the treeline, a surreal scene unfolded. Thousands of points of light glistened from countless little towns and ranches in the valleys below and from remote areas on the plains of Colorado. A full moon shone so brightly that it was actually possible to follow the trail in the moonlight, and most hikers switched off their headlamps. Even so, a string of bobbing headlamps could be seen marching up the trail far below. As we climbed higher, the eastern sky filled with soft shades of pink and cobalt, signaling a glorious dawn. It was a beautiful and unforgettable sight.

I reached the Boulder Field Campsites at 6 a.m., just as the mountain was beginning to glow from sunrise. I sat down among the rocks for a rest and a snack, and suddenly realized how cold I was. The exercise of climbing the trail had kept my core body temperature up, but my fingers were so numb that I couldn't open a package of granola or even zip up my jacket. It was a little alarming. The recognizable fea-

Hikers on the summit of Longs Peak

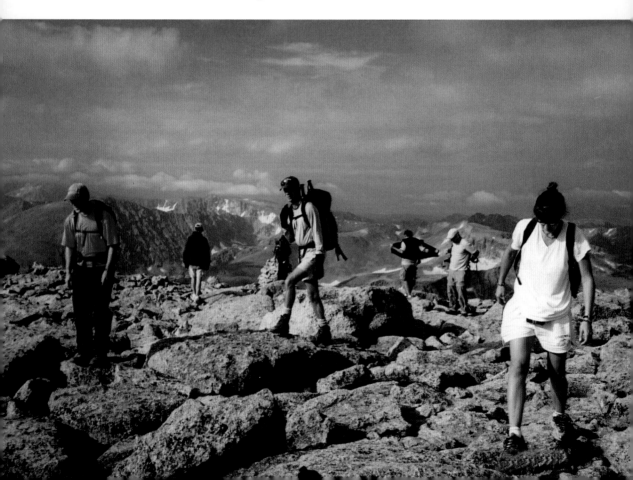

ture known as the "Keyhole" on the ridge above was already bathed in sunlight, so I decided to climb up to the warmth of the sun.

Within an hour, I reached the Keyhole. The Agnes Vaille Memorial Hut, a little stone shelter dedicated to two mountaineers who froze to death here in 1925, was tucked just beneath the Keyhole. After warming in the sun beside the hut, I started traversing the ledges on the still shady west face of Longs Peak. At the end of the traverse I looked up the feature called the Trough, and my jaw dropped. It seemed like hundreds of hikers were in the Trough, all inching slowly upward toward a small notch in the ridgeline above. I couldn't remember ever seeing as many hikers in one place—like scores of lemmings on some mysterious migration. I joined the rest of the lemmings and started up the Trough.

The Trough was steep, and the hoard of hikers above caused some debris to fall. At the top of the Trough I waited my turn to climb a slick granite slab to the beginning of the Narrows. The Narrows was an exposed and spectacular ledge system on the southeast face of Longs Peak. Below were Sand Beach Lake, where John Wesley Powell camped in 1868, and a large, gray fire-damaged area known as the Ouzel Burn. At the end of the Narrows, I came to a long granite slab leading to the summit, where I finally stepped on top. The broad summit of Longs Peak is as big as a football field, and it's a good thing, too, as I was in the company of at least a hundred other climbers. I had a welcome rest and took my turn in the queue to stand on the little rock that marks the highest point on the mountain. I started back down the Homestretch, and the only delay came at one point on the Narrows where only one person could pass at a time, and there was considerable negotiation for passage between those coming up and those going down.

By the time I reached the Keyhole, I was feeling the strain of a long, hard day, and it was only 11 a.m.! I had lunch at Boulder Field Campsite in the company of three very well-fed marmots. Back on the trail, I was happy to be off the tiring boulders at last and back on a flat path. The rest of the descent went well, although I was exhausted when I reached the trailhead. The entire hike had taken me nearly 12 hours.

My Longs Peak hike met all my expectations. It was challenging but also inspiring and intensely satisfying. The climb was an exhilarating alpine experience, made nonetheless magnificent by sharing it with many other companions, some of whom I became acquainted with during our hours together on the trail. Longs Peak is a true Rocky Mountain classic.

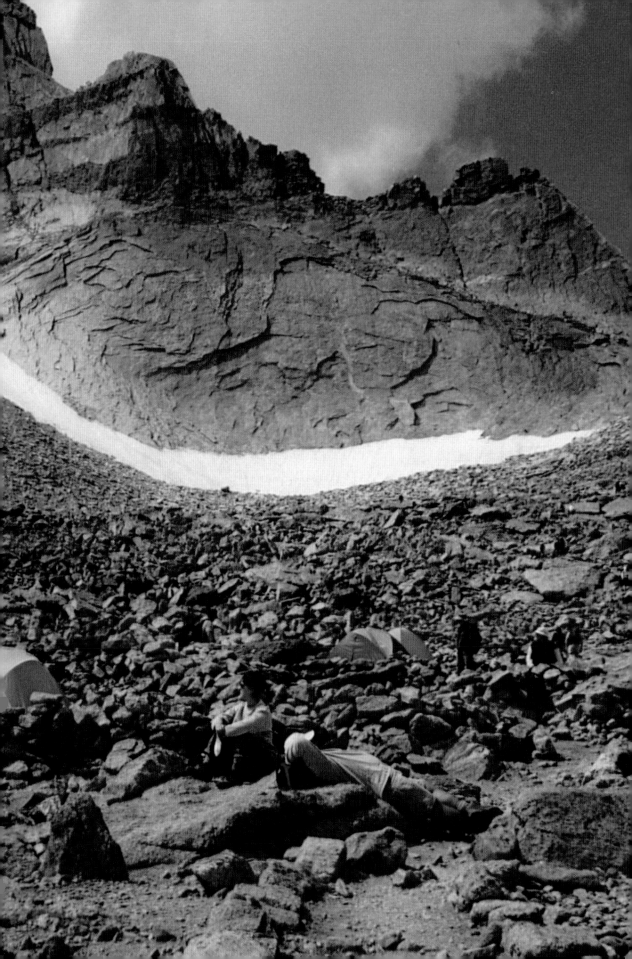

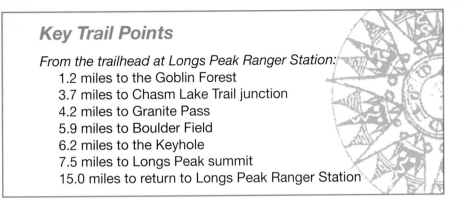

Key Trail Points

From the trailhead at Longs Peak Ranger Station:
- 1.2 miles to the Goblin Forest
- 3.7 miles to Chasm Lake Trail junction
- 4.2 miles to Granite Pass
- 5.9 miles to Boulder Field
- 6.2 miles to the Keyhole
- 7.5 miles to Longs Peak summit
- 15.0 miles to return to Longs Peak Ranger Station

DIRECTIONS TO TRAILHEAD AND TRAIL ROUTE

To reach the trailhead, drive to Longs Peak Ranger Station, 1 mile west of CO 7 and about 9 miles south of Estes Park, Colorado. The Ranger Station is open daily during the summer from 8 a.m. until 4:30 p.m. The parking lot at the Ranger Station fills up early on busy summer weekends, and the roadside is often parked full far down toward CO 7. For latecomers, this congestion can add hundreds of yards to an already long and arduous hike. But there is an even better reason to start early; severe afternoon thunderstorms are common in summer and have, on occasion, been fatal. Hikers usually start before 3 a.m. in order to be off the summit before noon. Sign the register at the trailhead before starting up the trail, and be sure to have a headlamp or flashlight.

About 1 mile from the trailhead, enter the krummholz (known here as Goblins Forest) region of gnarled and stunted trees that manage to survive the violent weather near treeline. Once above treeline the lights of distant ranches and villages become visible below but soon fade with the coming of dawn. The trail gradually ascends past the junction to Columbine Falls and Chasm Lake and on to Granite Pass at 12,080 feet—4.2 miles from the trailhead.

After about 6 miles on the trail, enter Boulder Field at 12,800 feet. Up to this point the trail is straightforward and well maintained, but here the trail gradually deteriorates to boulder-hopping and scrambling. Nine backcountry campsites are available in Boulder Field, but overnight camping will not be of interest for the determined day-hiker.

Longs Peak from the
Boulder Field

From Boulder Field, scramble west to the Keyhole—an overhanging notch in the ridgeline high above at about 13,000 feet—then traverse south across a steep ledge system on the west face. Ascend the Trough, a steep gully at the end of the traverse that has the highest accident rate on the route. A steep step at the top of the Trough is the crux of the climb. Next, traverse a narrow ledge system called the Narrows. The Narrows is the most exposed and precarious part of the route, and can be especially congested on busy summer weekends. A large rock below the Narrows is appropriately named the Hearse. The Homestretch is the final rocky slab leading upward to the summit. The route from the Keyhole to the summit is marked with yellow and red bull's-eyes painted on the rocks.

Return to the trailhead at Longs Peak Ranger Station by retracing the ascent route in reverse.

The "Keyhole" and Agnes Vaille Memorial Hut

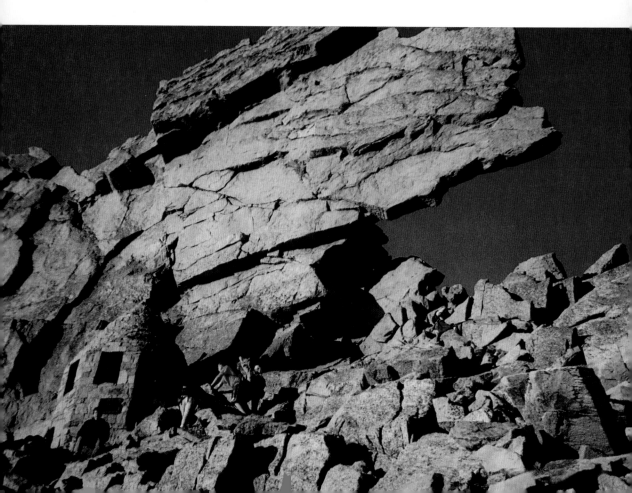

WEATHER AND WILDLIFE

In late July, August, and part of September, the Keyhole Route is generally free of snow and can be climbed without technical equipment. From about mid-September until mid-July, Longs Peak should not be attempted by anyone without crampons and an ice ax and the skill to use them. Afternoon thunderstorms are common on Longs Peak. Be aware of sudden changes in the weather and turn back to the safety of the lower elevations at the first sign of a storm. Hypothermia can occur on Longs Peak any time of year. Fall in Rocky Mountain National Park is generally dry, with crisp air and clear skies, but early snowstorms may also occur. Trail Ridge Road usually closes in mid-October.

Elk, bighorn sheep, moose, mule deer, and pronghorn antelope are common in Rocky Mountain National Park. Yellow-bellied marmots and ground squirrels are sure to be seen by anyone climbing Longs Peak. Pikas are less visible, but their high-pitched squeak will almost surely be heard above treeline.

LODGING AND CAMPING

Numerous options for lodging and services are located just outside the park in Estes Park, Colorado.

There are five drive-in campgrounds in Rocky Mountain National Park. Moraine Park and Aspenglen Campgrounds accept reservations at (877) 444-6777 or at **www.recreation.gov.** Longs Peak Campground, located near the trailhead, has only 26 campsites and is operated on a first-come, first-serve basis. Campground fees range from $14 to $20 per night. Overnight permits for camping at the Boulder Field on the trail can be obtained from Ranger Stations, or by calling the Backcountry Park Office at (970) 586-1242.

FEES AND CONTACTS

The entrance fee for Rocky Mountain National Park is $20 per day for a seven-day pass.

For more information, write to Backcountry Office, Rocky Mountain National Park, Estes Park, CO 80517. Phone (970) 586-1242 to check conditions on Longs Peak. The park's Web site is **www.nps.gov/romo.**

18 CHICAGO BASIN

Location: *San Juan Mountains, CO*
Distance: *14 miles*
Elevation Extremes: *8,210 to 11,240 feet*
Total Elevation Gain: *3,050 feet*
Difficulty: *Very Strenuous*
USGS Maps: *Snowdon Peak 7.5-minute, Mountain View Crest 7.5-minute, Columbine Pass 7.5-minute*
Trailhead Coordinates: *N 37° 38' 26.0" W 107° 41' 30.0"*
UTM 13S 0262510 4169348 [WGS 84]

THE NEED FOR SPEED

Every year thousands of tourists thrill to take one of the most spectacularly scenic trips in America: the Durango & Silverton Narrow Gauge Railroad (D&SNGRR), a historic coal-fired, steam-powered train that runs through the heart of the San Juan Mountains in southwestern Colorado. The Denver and Rio Grande Railway originally constructed the line in 1881 and 1882 to exploit the silver and mineral riches of the San Juan Mountains. The train has been in continuous operation for 122 years, delighting passengers with its vintage locomotives and cars. The National Park Service designated the entire line as a National Historic Landmark in 1967, and in 2000 the Society of American Travel Writers named the D&SNGRR as one of the Top Ten Train Journeys in the World.

Today, most passengers ride the train 45 miles from Durango to Silverton and return, passing through the spectacular Animas River Canyon. Few realize that, if requested, the train will stop at inaccessible trailheads where hikers can disembark. The most popular destination for these hikers is the Chicago Basin, a stunning alpine cirque ringed by four major peaks more than 14,000 feet high, as well as seven other distinct summits more than 13,000 feet high.

My stress level was already high that late July morning, knowing I was about to attempt a difficult hike. I would be covering 14 miles round-trip and gaining more than 3,000 feet on a tight timetable: The train would depart Durango at 9 a.m., hit the Needleton Trailhead stop mid-morning, and would be back in Needleton for a late-afternoon return to Durango. That meant just a few hours to make the hike.

So imagine my shock when I boarded the train and found my seat

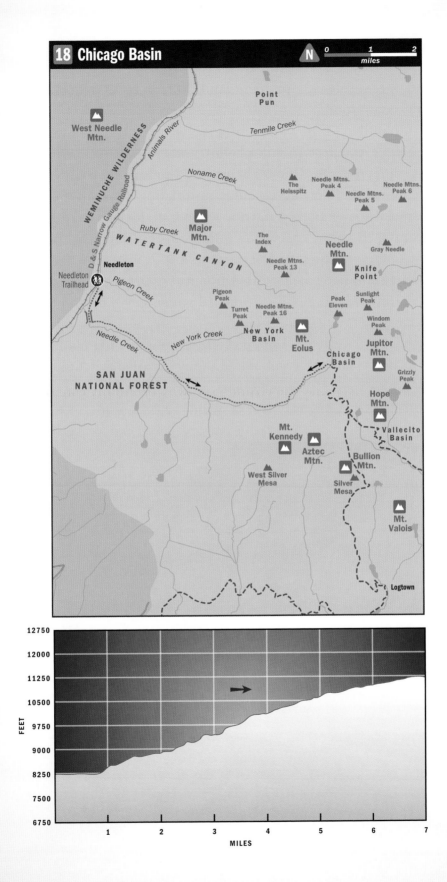

18 Chicago Basin

N   0   1   2
      miles

Point
Pun

West Needle
Mtn.

WEMINUCHE WILDERNESS

Animas River

Tenmile Creek

Noname Creek

The
Heisspitz

Needle Mtns.
Peak 4

Needle Mtns.
Peak 5

Needle Mtns.
Peak 6

Ruby Creek

Major
Mtn.

The
Index

Needle
Mtn.

Gray Needle

D & S Narrow Gauge Railroad

WATERTANK CANYON

Needle Mtns.
Peak 13

Knife
Point

Needleton

Needleton
Trailhead

Pigeon Creek

Pigeon
Peak

Turret
Peak

Needle Mtns.
Peak 16

New York
Basin

Mt.
Eolus

Peak
Eleven

Sunlight
Peak

Windom
Peak

Chicago
Basin

Jupitor
Mtn.

Grizzly
Peak

Needle Creek

New York Creek

SAN JUAN
NATIONAL FOREST

Hope
Mtn.

Vallecito
Basin

Mt.
Kennedy

Aztec
Mtn.

Bullion
Mtn.

West Silver
Mesa

Silver
Mesa

Mt.
Valois

Logtown

12750
12000
11250
10500
9750
9000
8250
7500
6750

FEET

1   2   3   4   5   6   7

MILES

already occupied. When I checked my ticket, my jaw dropped. It was for June 21—not July 21! Fortunately, I had time for a quick trip to the ticket window to resolve the problem. And I was in luck—rebooking my seat on this same train.

The train pulled puffing and shrieking out of Durango and followed along US 550 for the first 15 miles before entering the Animas River Canyon. At milepost 469.5 the train crossed the famous High Line, considered one of the most spectacular railroading views in the world. Here the tracks snake along a narrow ledge high above the Animas River (meaning "River of Lost Souls"). Passengers gasped at the sheer drop, and camera shutters clicked in rapid fire. It was easy to see why these old narrow gauge tracks, only three feet apart, were never converted to a standard gauge line. Standard gauge never could have made the sharp curves of the High Line.

At Needleton Trailhead, I hopped off for my carefully planned hike, with each little bridge and creek noted in my detailed schedule. I would

The D&SNGRR Train in Animas River Canyon

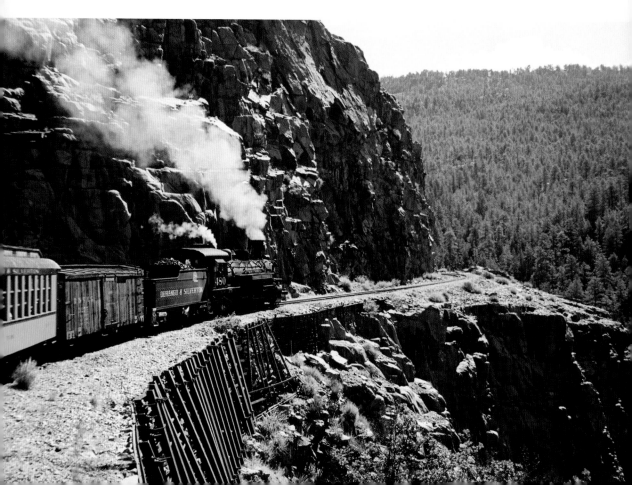

have to push hard, with little or no time to rest, to complete this trek in a single day. If I missed the last train at the Needleton stop, I would—literally—be up a creek. I had told my wife and daughter, Mary Fran and Jenny, that if I did miss it, they could pick me up in Purgatory, Colorado, at 10 p.m. It would take me that long, in the late, darkening afternoon, to hike the extra 9 miles out of the canyon. But this did not seem like a good option. I have always been skeptical of speed hiking, but the vision of Purgatory, pun intended, would surely keep me going.

I crossed the footbridge across the Animas River and turned south toward Needle Creek. The first part of the trail was smooth and flat, so I jogged a little to gain time. I came to a small footbridge at Needle Creek and began the long climb toward Chicago Basin. The trail climbed steadily on the north side of the creek, with occasional lovely views of Mountain View Crest to the south. Unfortunately, I had little time to pause and appreciate the scenery. I pushed my pace for the next 6 miles and was pleased to gain a little time on my schedule at each waypoint: first 8 minutes, then 12 minutes, then 15 minutes. I arrived panting at the head of Chicago Basin at 2:10 p.m., 20 minutes ahead of my schedule, so I took a few minutes to appreciate my surroundings.

The basin before me lived up to my lofty expectations. Four 14,000-foot peaks—Mount Eolus, North Eolus, Sunlight Peak, and Windom Peak—surrounded me. Numerous other slightly lesser peaks completed the scene. The open meadows were carpeted with a profusion of wild-flowers, including giant blue columbine. Two mountain goats, a nanny and her kid, walked casually through the meadow as a hiker grazed his pack llamas along the stream below. It was a scene I would have liked to savor a while longer, but, unfortunately, my schedule did not allow me to linger. There are those who enjoy the challenge and competition of speed hiking, but I was finding that it was detracting from my enjoy-ment of the hike. Thunder rolling through the peaks and a brief rain shower added to my haste, and I started down the trail.

I felt sure that meeting my schedule would be relatively easy going downhill, but I was dismayed to find that I was losing ground at each waypoint. Wherever the trail was smooth and the grade was gentle, I jogged a little. But I was still having trouble keeping up. As I neared the trailhead, I became more and more anxious. What if the train was early?

Fortunately, I reached the Needleton flag stop eight minutes ahead of schedule, and breathed a sigh of relief. Mary Fran and Jenny were

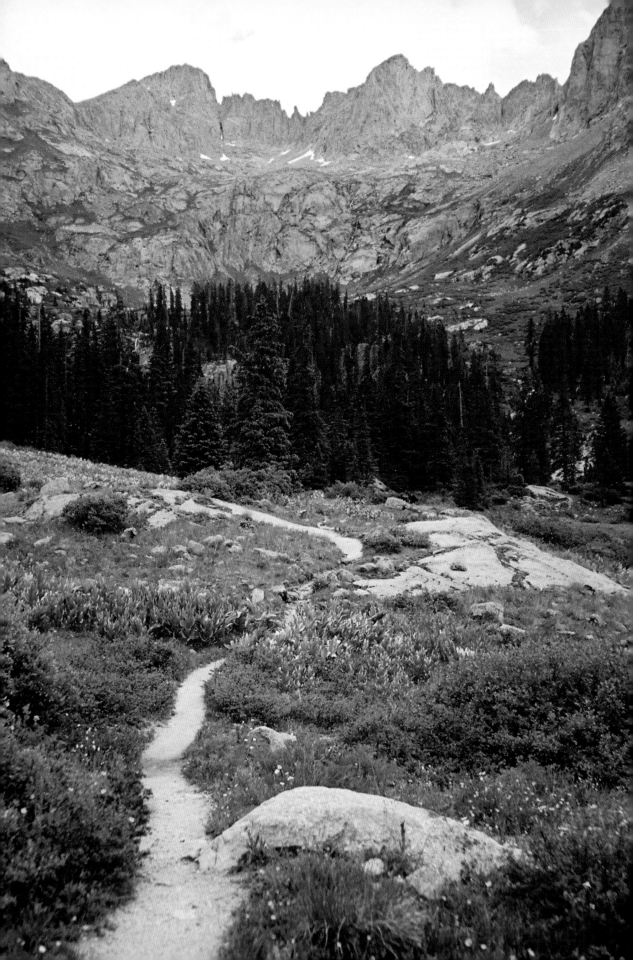

anxiously riding that same train after a day of gift-shopping in Silverton, and the conductor didn't help their frame of mind when he told them that it doesn't stop at Needleton. But there I was, standing on the tracks waving my arms across my knees, the signal to stop. The conductor would either have to stop or risk running me over.

The train did stop, of course, and I climbed aboard for the leisurely ride to Durango. With another passage along the High Line through Animas River Canyon, I had completed my memorable journey back in time on the vintage D&SNGRR and up to a fantastic alpine basin all in the same day. However, I did not particularly enjoy the need for speed on this hike. It certainly would have been a more pleasurable journey at a more leisurely pace. But for those who enjoy a demanding challenge in a spectacular setting, the hike to Chicago Basin in a single day cannot be matched.

Key Trail Points

From the Needleton Trailhead at milepost 483.3:
  0.8 miles to Needle Creek footbridge
  2.5 miles to New York Creek
  7.0 miles to Chicago Basin
  14.0 miles to return to Needleton Trailhead

DIRECTIONS TO TRAILHEAD AND TRAIL ROUTE

The Needleton Trailhead is a scheduled whistle-stop on the historic Durango & Silverton Narrow Gauge Railroad at milepost 483.8. The first train that will stop at Needleton leaves Durango at 9 a.m., and normally runs from mid-May to Mid-October. The 9 a.m. train is scheduled to stop at Needleton at 11:32 a.m., but the train will not stop unless the conductor is informed of the need to disembark. Earlier trains are scheduled during the summer season, but those will not stop at Needleton.

From the whistle-stop at Needleton, cross the Animas River on a footbridge and walk downriver on good trail to a footbridge across Needle Creek. Just before the footbridge, turn left up Needle Creek on Forest Trail 504 toward Chicago Basin. This trail climbs steeply 6.2 miles to Chicago Basin at 11,240 feet.

The trail in Chicago Basin

From Chicago Basin, return to the Needleton whistle-stop on the D&SNGRR by the same route. The day-hiker to Chicago Basin must carefully plan the itinerary and turn back short of the goal if necessary. Missing the last train back to Durango is not an option. The procedure for flagging a train is to stand beside the tracks and wave your arms across your knees. Once on the train, breathe a sigh of relief and enjoy the ride back to Durango.

The last train to Durango departs Silverton at 3:30 p.m. and arrives in Needleton at about 4:30 p.m. *Note: Train schedules show that this train does not stop at Needleton, but train personnel confirm that the last train will, and often does, stop to pick up hikers.* Even so, this only leaves a little less than five hours for the demanding hike to the Chicago Basin and back. The hiker must therefore average a pace in excess of 2.8 miles per hour, which, for this trail, probably cannot be done without at least a little jogging. Sticking to the published schedule would allow about four hours for the hike, which would not be possible for many—who would want to go partway only.

Blue Columbine in the Chicago Basin

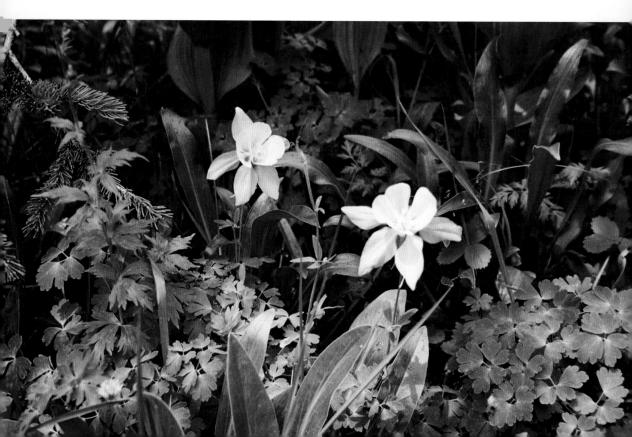

The last train to Durango only runs from the first week of June until mid-August (check the latest schedules on the Web site listed below). This leaves a fairly narrow window when this hike can be done in a single day. Winter snow remains deep in the Needle Mountains through mid-July, so the Chicago Basin can only be day-hiked from mid-July until mid-August.

An obvious alternative is to pack up the trail and overnight in the basin, and many hikers consider this attractive. For those who do not like to carry a heavy pack long distances—as I do not—another alternative would be to pack a tent, sleeping bag, and overnight gear, and leave the pack at Needleton or at one of the campsites along Needle Creek about 1 mile south of the trailhead. The return train to Durango can then be flagged the next day.

WEATHER AND WILDLIFE

As with any high-altitude hike in the Rocky Mountains, weather may change rapidly and can be extreme, even in summer. Be prepared for thunderstorms, hail, or even snow. Daily temperatures can range from warm and pleasant to cold and uncomfortable.

Animals common in the high country include mountain goats, bighorn sheep, marmots, and pikas. A population of elk winters in the Animas River Valley and grazes in the high country in summer. Less commonly seen are bobcats, mountain lions, and black bears.

LODGING AND CAMPING

A primitive backcountry campground is available along Needle Creek about 1 mile south of Needleton. A variety of private campgrounds, lodging, and services are available in and around Durango, Colorado.

FEES AND CONTACTS

Tickets for the D&SNGRR should be purchased several weeks in advance. Reservations can be made online at **www.railsnw.com,** or by phone at (503) 292-5055 or (800) 717-0108. The cost for a round-trip is $81 per adult and $49 per child ages 4–11 (plus taxes and fees), whether the destination is Silverton or a trailhead along the way.

19 HIGHLINE TRAIL–LOOP TRAIL

Location: *Glacier National Park, MT*
Distance: *11.1 miles*
Elevation Extremes: *4,310 to 7,020 feet*
Total Elevation Gain: *910 feet*
Difficulty: *Strenuous*
USGS Maps: *Logan Pass 7.5-minute, Many Glacier 7.5-minute, Ahern Pass 7.5-minute*
Trailhead Coordinates: *N 48° 41' 47.0" W 113° 43' 3.2"*
UTM 12U 0300047 5397274 [WGS 84]

A GRIZZLY ENCOUNTER

"Don't worry," I said. "This trail is so heavily traveled, the bears won't come anywhere near it!" I tried to sound confident. My wife, Mary Fran, was concerned about a possible encounter with a grizzly. It didn't help her frame of mind that an *Ursus arctos horribilis* sow had actually mauled two of our friends 12 years ago while hiking in Glacier National Park. Sue and Mitch still carry dreadful scars from that horrific ordeal. Nor did it inspire confidence that I had just encountered my first grizzlies, a mother and two cubs, the day before near Many Glacier Lake. But I had been anticipating hiking the famed Highline Trail for so long that I would not be deterred. After all, how likely would it be to meet a grizzly bear on the trail?

The plan was simple. I would drop Mary Fran off at Logan Pass on Going-to-the-Sun Road, then drive 7 miles west to leave our car at the Loop, which would be the end of our hike. I would then hitchhike back to Logan Pass to start our hike at the trailhead. The "Crown of the Continent" Highline Trail runs almost flat along the base of the famous Garden Wall for 7.6 miles to the Granite Park Chalet. We wanted to stay overnight at this national historic landmark hotel, reached only by trail, in the panoramic and pristine wilderness of Glacier National Park. We could then walk 3.5 miles down the Loop Trail to the car the next morning. It was a perfect plan, if only the bears would cooperate!

It was July, perhaps a little early in the season for this hike, but this day the weather was perfect. I dropped Mary Fran off at Logan Pass before noon and drove down to the Loop. I could have easily

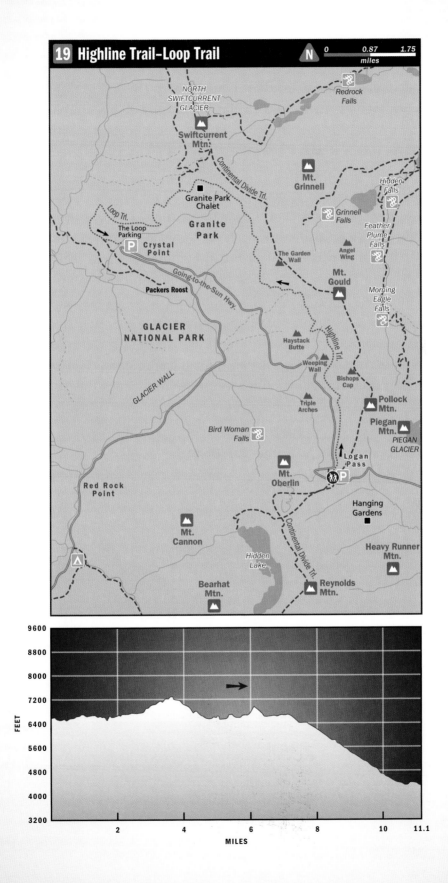

19 Highline Trail–Loop Trail

N   0   0.87   1.75
miles

NORTH SWIFTCURRENT GLACIER

Redrock Falls

Swiftcurrent Mtn.

Continental Divide Trl.

Mt. Grinnell

Hidden Falls

Granite Park Chalet

Grinnell Falls

Loop Trl.

Feather Plume Falls

The Loop Parking

Granite Park

Crystal Point

The Garden Wall

Angel Wing

Mt. Gould

Morning Eagle Falls

Going-to-the-Sun Hwy.

Packers Roost

GLACIER NATIONAL PARK

Haystack Butte

Highline Trl.

Weeping Wall

Bishops Cap

GLACIER WALL

Triple Arches

Pollock Mtn.

Piegan Mtn.

PIEGAN GLACIER

Bird Woman Falls

Logan Pass

Red Rock Point

Mt. Oberlin

Hanging Gardens

Mt. Cannon

Heavy Runner Mtn.

Hidden Lake

Continental Divide Trl.

Bearhat Mtn.

Reynolds Mtn.

FEET

9600
8800
8000
7200
6400
5600
4800
4000
3200

2   4   6   8   10   11.1

MILES

waited for the next park shuttle bus to come along, but I was in a hurry and put out my thumb. A few cars went by before an elderly woman in an old Jeep picked me up and took me back to the top of the pass. A magnificent bighorn ram was strolling through the parking lot as I thanked the woman for the lift. The day was off to a good start. Mary Fran and I ate lunch in the Logan Pass Visitor Center, walked across the highway, and started down Highline Trail.

The trail exceeded my expectations right from the start. Mountain goats grazed along the way completely unconcerned by our presence. Bighorn sheep were a little more wary as they looked down from the rocks above. At times the trail was cut into a near-vertical rock face, with nerve-racking drops to the meadows below. And the crowning glory was an unexpected profusion of wildflowers. Red Indian paintbrush, glacier lilies, arctic willows, sky pilots, yellow arnicas, and groundsels dazzled our eyes at every turn. And most striking of all were fields of thousands of distinctive beargrass blossoms, the unofficial flower of Glacier Park. First named by explorers Lewis and Clark, beargrass is an important browse for deer, elk, and bighorn sheep. Only four days

The Highline Trail and Going-to-the-Sun Road
near Logan Pass

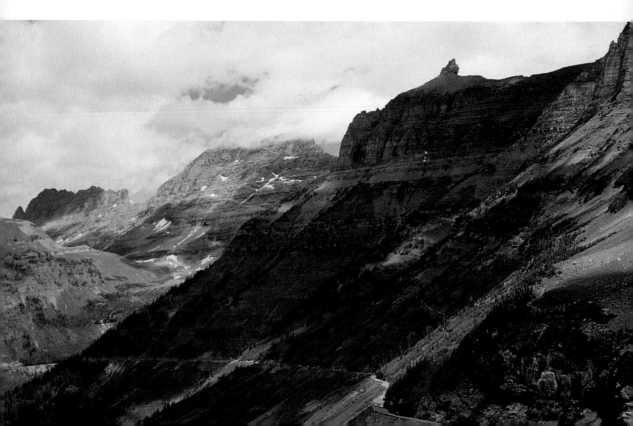

before, we had hiked Mount Rainier's Spray Park Trail—reputed to have the best wildflower display on the planet—but the flowers on Highline Trail were every bit as spectacular, if not more so. Two professional photographers were traveling the trail at about the same pace as we were, and they were literally giddy with the show.

After two hours on the trail, we came to a climb of about 200 feet to reach a pass behind Haystack Butte. This was the biggest ascent on the trail, and it was gentle enough, but the final grade was covered in snow, making it slippery and a little tiring. Haystack Butte was the halfway point, and from here the trail ambled easily through meadows and talus slopes toward Granite Park Chalet.

We rounded a bend in the trail to see the photographers eagerly pointing up the slope, and there he was—a large male grizzly bear foraging in the meadow above the trail. He seemed harmless enough, about 200 yards away, and totally focused on his digging. Mary Fran was not pleased, but we watched the bear for a while, took a couple of pictures, and then headed on toward the chalet. I glanced back to notice the photographers walking briskly in our direction, and looked up the slope to see the grizzly lumbering down toward us. We picked up the pace. The next time I looked back, the bear was on the trail about 40 yards behind us, and walking swiftly in our direction. Mary Fran was more than alarmed and kicked it into a hiking gear I didn't know she had!

As we neared the chalet, a boy and two girls approached walking toward the bear, which was then out of sight around a bend. Despite my warning, the boy assumed a macho air and continued on. "Don't worry," he said. "We'll be OK!" But as soon as they rounded the bend and saw the rapidly approaching bear, they beat a hasty retreat. We were now seven people scurrying toward the safety of the chalet. We all reached it together breathless but otherwise unharmed. We watched the grizzly amble to the meadow far above. Was he stalking us or simply going our way on the trail? To this day I still don't know.

The Granite Park Chalet itself is a jewel set in the crown of the continent, and one of the great historic lodges of the national parks. Built out of native stone and timber in 1915 and 1916 by the Great Northern Railway, Granite Park Chalet is one of only two backcountry chalets in Glacier to survive. Perched on an outcrop of granite, and with a spectacular, expansive vista of the surrounding mountains, Granite Park Chalet is truly a one-of-a-kind experience. Its grand panoramic vista drops sharply to Bear Valley then ascends to Heavens Peak, Longfellow Peak, and Wolf Gun Mountain. It dazzled us as we sat on the front porch.

After marveling at the view, we went inside to register with the chalet host. He showed us to our room and gave us linens, which cost an extra $30 ($15 per person) but was worth it since it eliminated the need to carry sleeping bags. It was the ultimate room with a view. We were about to schedule a time to use the kitchen when the leader of a large group said, "We have plenty of food. Why not eat with us?" So we added good company to an already wonderful journey.

After supper we went out to watch a glorious sunset over Heavens Peak. At dark we went in to sit by the fire and listen to our host, who used to be a Glacier park ranger, tell bear stories that were both humorous and horrific. He said the bear that followed us was becoming a nuisance bear around the chalet, and would need to "be taken care of." This meant that park rangers would shoot it with rubber bullets, hoping to hurt it just enough so that it would shun human presence and move on. Later that night when I needed to get up and make my way to the latrine, I couldn't help wondering if the bear was out there waiting for me in the dark.

The next morning, Mary Fran and I were up early and hiked down the Loop Trail, which descended through an area ravaged by fire in 2003. Today this clear land is a favorite browse for deer, and we saw several. The hike down to the Loop took an easy two hours, and our morning ended with a fine breakfast at Lake McDonald Lodge, another one of the classics built by the Great Northern Railway in the 1920s.

The combination of the Highline Trail and the Granite Park Chalet, not to mention our grizzly encounter, made this adventure one of the most memorable of my life. In my mind, the wildlife, flowers, and constant vistas along Highline Trail are unmatched by any other trail in the Rocky Mountain West.

DIRECTIONS TO TRAILHEAD AND TRAIL ROUTE

The "Crown of the Continent" Highline Trail begins at Logan Pass on the Going-to-the-Sun Road at 6,646 feet and leads north along the base of the Garden Wall, a dramatic rock face towering high above the trail. Mountain goats and bighorn sheep roam freely on the green slopes, and a profusion of wildflowers grace the meadows. The trail climbs slightly to pass behind Haystack Butte, and then continues on to Granite Park Chalet. A

Key Trail Points

From the trailhead at Logan Pass:
  3.5 miles to Haystack Butte
  6.4 miles to Grinnell Glacier Overlook Trail junction
  7.6 miles to Granite Park Chalet
  11.1 miles to the Loop

diversion to Grinnell Glacier Overlook, 6.4 miles from Logan Pass, is well worth the effort if time permits. A full water bottle, insect repellant, and sunscreen will also be useful. A flashlight should be taken for night use.

From Granite Park Chalet, the Loop Trail descends 2,300 feet in 3.5 miles down to the small parking lot on the Going-to-the-Sun Road. Since the devastating 2003 fire, the slope has filled with new undergrowth, extensive wildflower displays, and open vistas. Deer commonly browse in the meadows below the chalet.

Mary Fran on the porch of the Granite Park Chalet

WEATHER AND WILDLIFE

Weather on the west side of the divide is temperate but temperamental in July and August, with temperatures ranging from 29° to 80°F. Evenings are usually cool, and the buildings are not heated, so warm clothing is recommended. Rain gear should always be carried to cope with sudden rain or snow squalls and thunderstorms. Snow will be encountered on the trail before mid-July.

Grizzly bears are the most famous and fearsome inhabitants of the park. Unlike some black bears, grizzlies are not predatory in nature, but they will fiercely defend their territory and their young. Hikers have been seriously injured, maimed, and even killed by grizzlies in Glacier Park. Do not surprise a bear. Announce your presence by singing or talking loudly and often. Bears will move away if they hear people coming. Bear bells, now facetiously referred to as "dinner bells," invite curiosity and are not as effective as once believed. Hiking alone is not recommended. If possible, hike in a group and stay together. Never approach a bear; they are exceptionally fast and you cannot outrun them.

In addition to grizzly bears, a wide variety of animals make their home in Glacier National Park. Mountain goats, bighorn sheep, deer, moose, elk, and coyotes are most visible. Grey wolves are making a comeback, and several wolf packs now range throughout the park. Bald eagles gathered in hundreds on the west side of the park until the salmon population collapsed in 1986, but they are still frequently seen.

LODGING AND CAMPING

Granite Park Chalet is typically open from about July 1 until early to mid-September. The chalet has 12 rooms, with sizes ranging from double occupancy to rooms for six, with single bunk beds in all of the rooms. Rooms are assigned at the time of reservation, and reservations must often be made months in advance. Rates are $85 per person and $73 for each additional person in the same room. Fresh linens can be reserved at the time of reservation for an additional $16 per person. No meals are served at the chalet, but a rustic kitchen is available for use by guests. A minimum of pans, pots, kitchen utensils, and cups are available for use. Limited refrigeration is available on a first-come, first-serve basis. Each guest must provide or disinfect his own water, with the nearest water source 0.25 miles away. Everything packed in must be packed out, including leftover food waste. The phone number for Granite Park Chalet is (888) 345-2649, or reservations can be made online at **www.graniteparkchalet.com/granite.html.**

There are several other historic lodges, as well as motels, within Glacier National Park. All are typically full in summer, so reservations should be made early with Glacier Park, Inc. at (406) 892-2525 or online at **www.glacierparkinc.com.** A variety of lodging and services convenient to this hike can also be found outside the west entrance to the park.

There are 13 campgrounds in Glacier National Park with a total of more than 1,000 campsites. Most convenient to this hike are the Sprague Creek, Avalanche, Rising Sun, and St. Mary campgrounds. Reservations can be made at St. Mary Campground at **www.recreation .gov,** with the others available on a first-come, first-serve basis. All of these campgrounds fill up early during July and August.

FEES AND CONTACTS
The entrance fee for Glacier National Park is $25 per vehicle ($15 in winter) for a seven-day pass.

Current information about weather, trail conditions, and bear activity can be obtained from Glacier National Park, PO Box 128, West Glacier, MT, 59936, or by phone at (406) 888-7800. The park's Web site is **www.nps.gov/glac,** or you can email the park at **glac_information @nps.gov.**

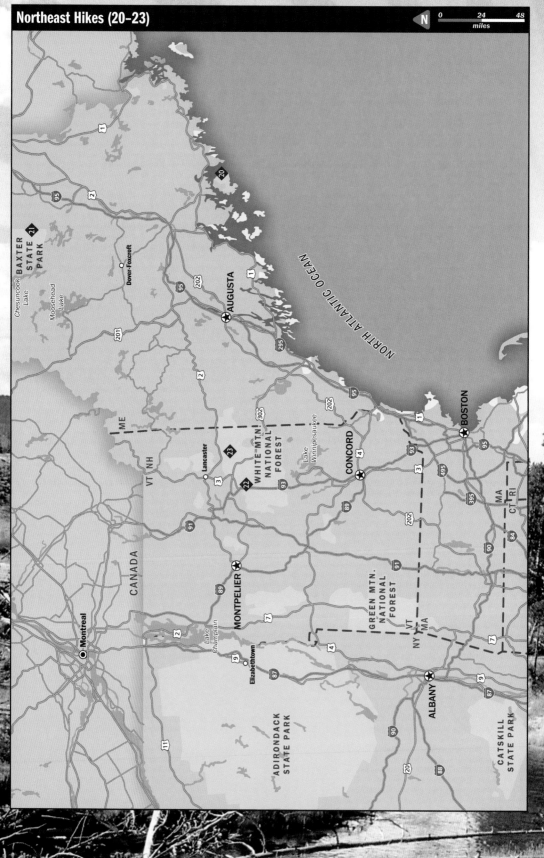

N

0   24   48
miles

NORTH ATLANTIC OCEAN

BAXTER STATE PARK 21

Chesuncook Lake

Moosehead Lake

Dover-Foxcroft

AUGUSTA

BOSTON

CONCORD

Lake Winnipesaukee

WHITE MTN. NATIONAL FOREST 22

23

Lancaster

ME
NH
VT

CANADA

Montreal

MONTPELIER

Lake Champlain

Elizabethtown

GREEN MTN. NATIONAL FOREST

NY
VT
MA

MA
CT
RI

ALBANY

ADIRONDACK STATE PARK

CATSKILL STATE PARK

1
95
2
201
202
95
2
295
95
302
202
3
93
89
202
91
91
90
395
84
7
93
9
87
2
7
4
9
87
90
111
20
88
20

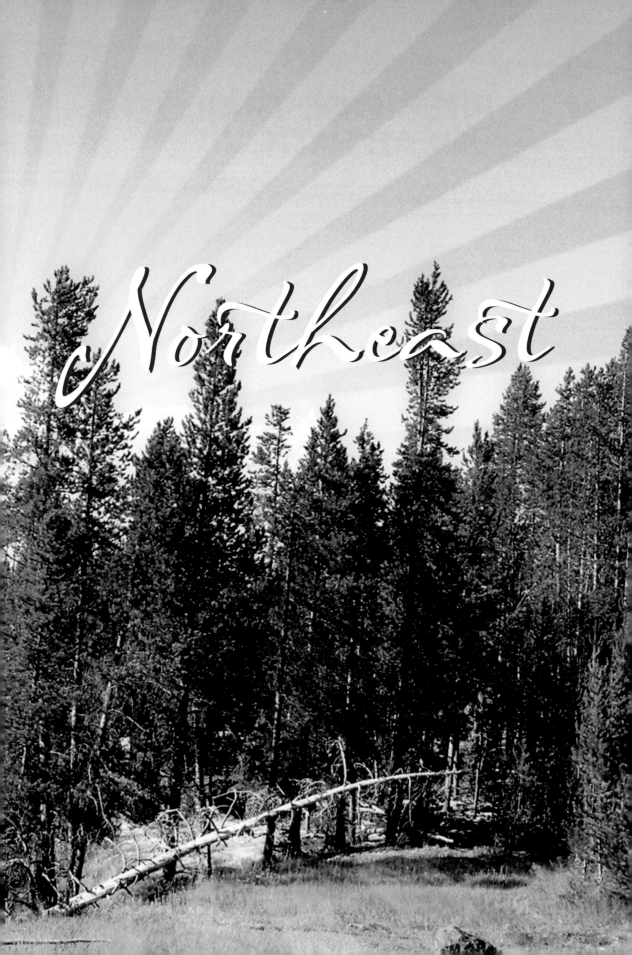

Northeast

20 PRECIPICE TRAIL TO OCEAN PATH

> **Location:** *Acadia National Park, Bar Harbor, ME*
> **Distance:** *5.6 miles*
> **Elevation Extremes:** *25 to 1,058 feet*
> **Total Elevation Gain:** *1,120 feet*
> **Difficulty:** *Moderate*
> **USGS Maps:** *Seal Harbor 7.5-minute*
> **Trailhead Coordinates:** *N 44° 20' 58.3" W 68° 11' 16.8"*
> *UTM 19T 0564730 4911010 [WGS 84]*

A FEARSOME REPUTATION

About midway along the rocky coast of Maine lies a unique island of sheer granite domes, tidal pools, and mud flats. Its tallest mountain is the highest point on the eastern seaboard of North America, and is the place where morning sunlight first strikes American soil (from October through March). The slopes of the mountains are cloaked in an incredible diversity of plants and wildlife, and are often shrouded in fog that enhances the beauty of the surrounding mountains and sea alike. This is Mount Desert Island of Acadia National Park, the first national park to be established east of the Mississippi River.

I had wanted to hike the Precipice Trail of Acadia National Park for a long time. It is possibly the most diverse—and precarious—of the maintained trails in the national park system. It ascends the sheer east face of Champlain Mountain by means of iron steps and ladders fixed to rock toward a summit 1,058 feet above the crashing surf. The fearsome reputation of Precipice Trail is well deserved.

I arrived at the trailhead for Precipice Trail midmorning in August and nearly missed my opportunity to experience this unique hike. Precipice Trail had been closed to protect nesting peregrine falcons up until only one week before my planned hike. So I was feeling lucky as I set off through the pitch-pine and burr-oak forest. I soon came to an angle in the cliff where iron steps had been fastened to a slightly overhanging granite face. I had a feeling that this was a test for things to come, as if to say, "If you have trouble here, don't even think about going higher!" After a strenuous pull-up, I continued on.

The angle of the trail increased, with handholds and occasional

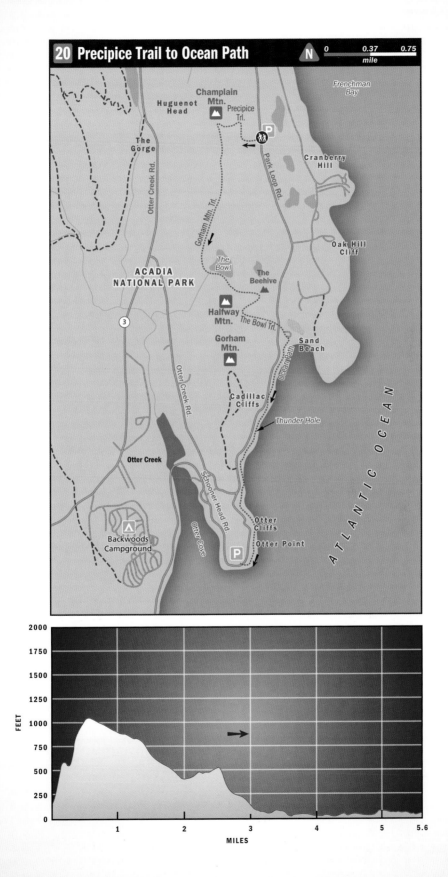

20 Precipice Trail to Ocean Path

N

0   0.37   0.75
mile

Frenchman Bay

Huguenot Head

Champlain Mtn.

Precipice Trl.

P

Cranberry Hill

The Gorge

Otter Creek Rd.

Park Loop Rd.

Oak Hill Cliff

Gorham Mtn. Trl.

ACADIA NATIONAL PARK

The Bowl

The Beehive

3

Halfway Mtn.

The Bowl Trl.

Sand Beach

Gorham Mtn.

Ocean Path

Otter Creek Rd.

Cadillac Cliffs

Thunder Hole

ATLANTIC OCEAN

Otter Creek

Schooner Head Rd.

Otter Cove

Otter Cliffs

Backwoods Campground

P

Otter Point

Elevation profile:

2000
1750
1500
1250
1000
750
500
250
0

FEET

1   2   3   4   5   5.6

MILES

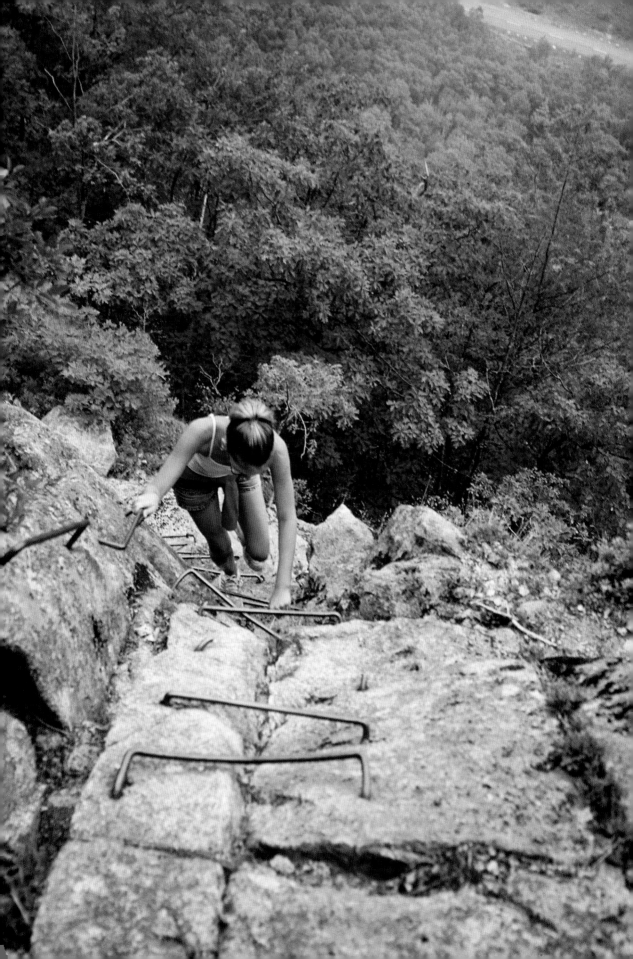

iron rods for steps, until I reached a long traverse to the right. Here I met two hikers going the other way. They were lost, and feared that they had missed a turn. I backtracked with them about 300 yards, losing some hard-won elevation in the process, and then went back up to find that the trail turned abruptly upward farther on. The "trail" got even steeper with more rungs and ladders leading ever upward. Finally I reached the open, craggy summit of Champlain Mountain at 11:50 a.m. Fog was shrouding the summit, lending a mysterious quality to the landscape. Farther to the west, about 500 feet higher, I could just make out Cadillac Mountain. Its summit was higher but was crowded with hoards of tourists cruising for a parking space. "This," I thought, "is the better spot."

After a brief lunch I headed down the trail toward Gorham Mountain and The Bowl. Gorham Mountain Trail was hard to follow across the rocky crest, and I had to backtrack twice to locate trail marks on the rocks. Somewhere on Gorham Mountain Trail, the silence was broken by the shrill sound of emergency sirens below. I later learned that a hiker had fallen from the cliffs along Ocean Path and had died before rescuers could reach him. There are several places along Precipice and Ocean Path trails where a slip could have fatal consequences.

After skirting a depression and small lake known as The Bowl, I took a short trail to the summit of The Beehive, which afforded another impressive view of Frenchman Bay. The scene from The Beehive was well worth another pause to take in the sweeping panorama of mountains and sea. From The Beehive I descended to Bowl Trail, and reached Sand Beach on the ocean by early afternoon. A couple of emergency vehicles were still present from the fatal hiking accident.

Switching to Ocean Path, the trail changed character dramatically from heavy woods and faraway rocky lookouts to an intimate marine setting. The fishy-sweet smell and the sound of waves lapping the rocks were constant reminders of the nearness of the sea. This coast is one of the world's most biologically productive areas, and the rocks were covered with barnacles, mussels, and dog whelks. I couldn't resist the temptation to explore a few tidal pools near the trail. The variety of life here, each adapted to its own specific tide level and exposure to the elements, has never failed to amaze me.

Precipice Trail climbs the Cliffs of Champlain Mountain.

The first part of Ocean Path followed along the Park Loop Road to Thunder Hole. A short side trail led to the brink of the hole, where waves usually funnel into the rocks and erupt in a spectacular show of sound and spray. Unfortunately, this day the waves were slight and the show was absent. Here I joined my wife, Mary Fran, who had decided to hike the Ocean Path from Otter Point to Sand Beach. She planned to catch the Island Explorer shuttle for a ride back to the car at Otter Point.

After Thunder Hole, Ocean Path diverged from the road and became even more delightful without the sounds and smell of traffic. I paused to take in the view from the Otter Cliffs, and reached the Otter Point parking area to wait for Mary Fran's arrival on the park shuttle. The entire hike had taken me a leisurely three-and-a-half hours. The most memorable quality of this hike was its variety: a precarious mountain climb on the notorious Precipice Trail, high mountain views, deep hardwood forests, sweeping seacoast vistas, and teeming marine life on the Ocean Path.

Ocean cliffs near Otter Point

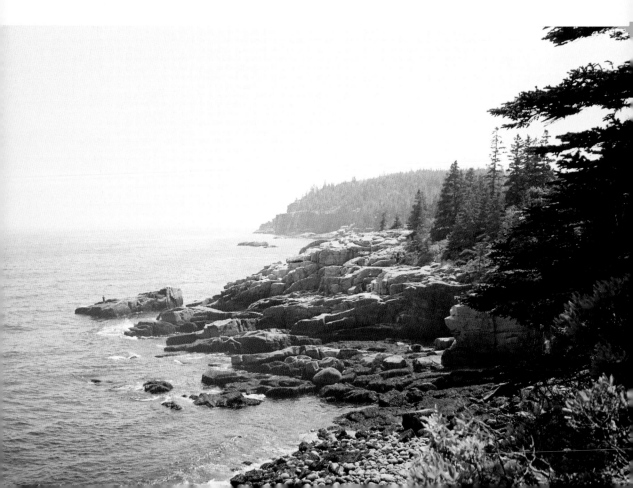

> ## Key Trail Points
>
> *From the trailhead on the Park Loop Road:*
>   0.8 miles to the summit of Champlain Mountain
>   2.4 miles to The Bowl
>   2.8 miles to The Beehive
>   3.7 miles to Sand Beach
>   4.4 miles to Thunder Hole
>   5.2 miles to Otter Cliffs
>   5.6 miles to Otter Cliffs parking area

DIRECTIONS TO TRAILHEAD AND TRAIL ROUTE

Acadia National Park is located 15 miles south of Ellsworth, Maine. The trailhead for the Precipice Trail is 3.5 miles south of Bar Harbor along the Park Loop Road. The Precipice Trail is not for the faint of heart. It begins innocently enough as it wanders through tranquil forest, but it steadily rises as you approach the granite cliffs. At times the "trail" climbs nearly vertical on iron steps and ladders, finally cresting on the rocky, barren summit of Champlain Mountain.

From the summit of Champlain Mountain, head south down Gorham Mountain Trail 1.6 miles toward The Bowl. The southern ridge of Champlain Mountain is exposed and rocky, and hikers must keep a sharp eye out for trail markers painted on the rocks. The Bowl cradles a secluded mountain lake where hikers often swim on warm summer days.

After skirting the southwestern shore of The Bowl, leave the Gorham Mountain Trail and bear left to the summit of the Beehive. The Beehive, 546 feet above sea level, is another exposed rocky knob with splendid views of Frenchman Bay and the surrounding mainland. Descend steeply 0.3 miles down the south side of the Beehive to intersect the Bowl Trail, and descend another 0.6 miles to Sand Beach on the coast.

From Sand Beach follow Ocean Path south to Thunder Hole, where waves funnel into a narrow cleft in the rock to rumble against the back wall of the chasm. Beyond Thunder Hole, Ocean Path veers away from the highway for lovely views of the rockbound coast of Maine. Another 0.8 miles brings you to Otter Cliffs, a high granite precipice overlooking the Atlantic Ocean and the Cranberry Islands to the south.

A final short trail leads to the parking area for Otter Point. This parking area, like the trailhead for the Precipice Trail, is on the route of the Island Explorer, a fare-free shuttle that circles the Park Loop

Road during the summer. Buses run frequently, so the shuttle can be used to return to a vehicle at the Precipice Trailhead, or hikers can choose to leave a vehicle at Otter Point and ride the shuttle first.

WEATHER AND WILDLIFE

The weather in Acadia is highly changeable anytime of year. Summer high temperatures average a comfortable 70° to 80°F, but fog is common. Spring and fall highs are 50° to 60°F. Winter lasts from November to April, and temperatures range from below 0° to 30°F. Annual snowfall averages 60 inches in Acadia.

A remarkable variety of wildlife can be seen in Acadia. The most common creature is the red squirrel, and its scolding chatter constantly breaks the silence of the forest. Larger mammals include the white-tailed deer, raccoons, and red foxes. Acadia supports a healthy population of coyotes, which feeds primarily on deer, raccoons, and small rodents. Otters play in lakes and beaver ponds, and gulls are seen everywhere along the shore. Eiders gather in huge rafts that stretch for hundreds of feet on the sea, and cormorants rest on ledges and rocks with their wings outstretched. It is now hard to imagine that at the turn of the century, gulls and other seabirds were almost extinct here. Eagles have also made a comeback, as has the peregrine falcon. The peregrine falcon's favorite nesting site is the cliffs of Champlain Mountain along the Precipice Trail. Four species of seals are found around Mount Desert Island. Harbor porpoises and dolphins can be seen farther offshore, and Orca whales are present in summer months. The small minke whale is often seen in Frenchman Bay, and humpback whales and right whales are also regular visitors. Finally, an astounding diversity of life can be seen in the tidal pools along the Ocean Path.

LODGING AND CAMPING

Many lodging options, as well as private campgrounds, are available in the nearby towns of Bar Harbor and Ellsworth and along Maine Highway 3 leading to the park.

There are two main park campgrounds on Mount Desert Island.
Blackwoods Campground is open
all year with reservations suggested   Thunder hole on the Ocean Walk

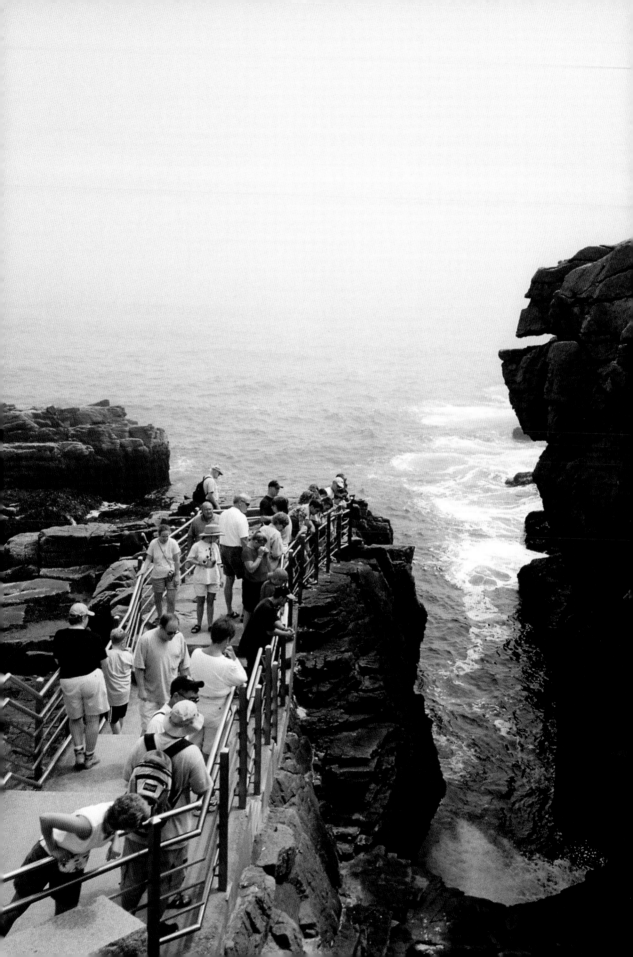

between May and October. Seawall Campground is operated in summer on a first-come, first-serve basis. Campsites are $20 per night (less in shoulder seasons). Raccoons are a particular problem in Acadia campgrounds, and food must be stored and disposed of correctly.

FEES AND CONTACTS

A $20 per vehicle entrance fee is charged for Acadia National Park from June 23 to early October. The fee is $10 in the shoulder seasons. The permit is good for seven days. The Island Explorer, the shuttle that circles the Park Loop Road, is free for visitors.

For more information, contact Acadia National Park, PO Box 177, Bar Harbor, ME 04609-0177, phone (207) 288-3338, or check the park's Web site at **www.nps.gov/acad**. Hikers should be sure to ask if Precipice Trail is open, as the trail is closed during early summer to protect peregrine falcons that nest high on the eastern cliffs of Champlain Mountain.

21 KNIFE EDGE OF MOUNT KATAHDIN

Location: *Baxter State Park, ME*
Distance: *10 miles*
Elevation Extremes: *1,495 to 5,267 feet*
Total Elevation Gain: *3,920 feet*
Difficulty: *Very Strenuous*
USGS Maps: *Katahdin Lake 7.5-minute, Mount Katahdin 7.5-minute*
Trailhead Coordinates: *N 45° 55' 12.1" W 68° 51' 27.9" UTM 19T 0511030 5085170 [WGS 84]*

"KETTE-ADENE," THE GREATEST MOUNTAIN

A huge mountain stands alone in the wild interior of north-central Maine. It is more reminiscent of rocky western peaks than any mountain I know east of the Mississippi. This granite giant, soaring high above the surrounding wilderness, is the most prominent feature of Maine. The Abenaki Indians knew it as Kette-Adene, meaning "greatest mountain." Today we know it as Mount Katahdin, the highest point in Maine and the northern terminus of the Appalachian Trail. Mount Katahdin is actually an enormous massif with several distinct summits surrounding a huge glacial cirque. Its summits include Pamola, Chimney Peak, South Peak, Hamlin Peak, the three Howe Peaks, and the highest summit, Baxter Peak, which rises to 5,267 feet above sea level.

Several trails may be taken to the Baxter Peak summit, but the most notorious is Knife Edge, a precarious exposed ridge that runs 1.1 miles from the Pamola summit to Baxter Peak. I first hiked Knife Edge about 25 years ago and was not surprised when my hiker's survey rated it as the second best hike in the Northeast. I was anxious to repeat this exciting climb, but I was a little concerned. The weather in early August, on the day of my adventure, was unsettled, and a quick exit from Knife Edge in bad weather is tricky business indeed.

Rick Givens, a friend of mine from Grove City College, picked me up at the Heritage Motor Inn in Millinocket at 4 a.m. We knew that the gatehouse at Togue Pond opened at 5 a.m. and that eager hikers would be waiting. No additional cars would be admitted after the Roaring Brook parking area was full. We drove through the Maine woods at predawn and arrived at the Togue Pond entrance in darkness 15

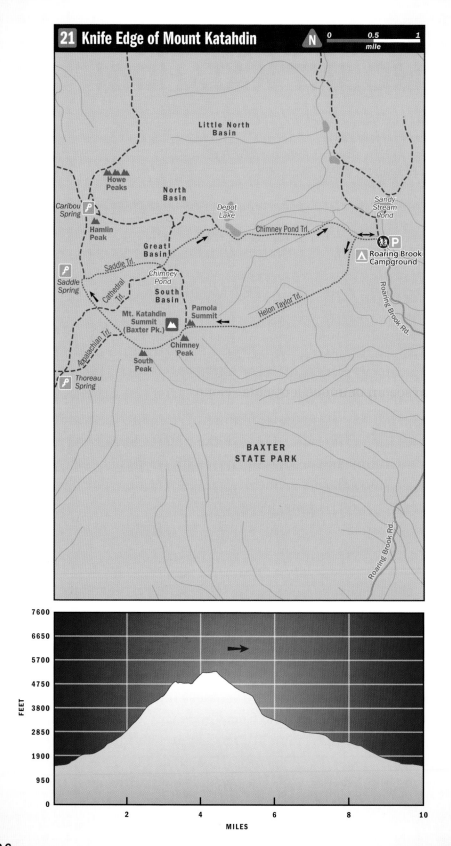

Knife Edge of Mount Katahdin

minutes before opening time. I was relieved to see only five cars at the gatehouse. There probably would have been more on a weekend.

Rick presented his driver's license, and we drove through the entrance. Rick lives in Millinocket, and the $8 entrance fee is waived for Maine residents. Always the complete outdoors couple, Rick and his wife moved to Maine after graduation and started a successful canoe livery and wilderness lodge business. Rick knows Mount Katahdin well and had been on Knife Edge several times before, though it always made even him nervous.

When we finally arrived at the Roaring Brook parking lot, I was shocked to see it about half full. People camping in the park overnight had already taken a serious toll on the parking-lot capacity. We packed up, signed the register, and were on our way up the Helon Taylor Trail by 5:40 a.m. The trail was harder than I remembered, and it takes a serious toll on the body. It was choked with boulders, sometimes requiring the use of our hands to climb higher, and was almost never flat.

We broke above treeline after approximately 2 miles, and I was alarmed to see an ominous lenticular cloud perched above Hamlin Peak. I had become well acquainted with lenticular clouds while climbing in Alaska, where these heralds of evil weather frequently sweep down the mountain and threaten to destroy everything in their path. But as we climbed higher, the cloud just seemed to dissolve. The weather was windy and dark, but it looked like it might hold off.

We arrived at the windswept summit of Pamola, with an elevation of 4,902 feet, at 8:30 a.m. A sign warned, "The Knife Edge, Baxter Peak 1.1 Miles, Do Not Hike in Threatening Weather." Good advice! The granite spine from here to Baxter Peak resembled a climb more than a hike, and Rick was not pleased, due to his anxiety about heights. The trail was especially precarious after the summit of Chimney Peak, only 0.1 mile from the summit of Pamola.

We climbed over South Peak—elevation 5,240 feet—at 9:40 a.m. and arrived at the Baxter Peak summit in the company of 17 other hikers at about 10 a.m. Dark clouds were whizzing over our heads, and the chilly temperature made us want to find shelter from the wind for an early lunch. The view across the sparkling lakes and the severe boreal forest of the Maine wilderness was awe-inspiring. An old weathered sign proclaimed, "Appalachian Trail—Springer Mountain, Georgia, 2,160 Miles." Shortly after we arrived, an elderly but obviously very fit hiker came trudging up the trail. With tears in his eyes, he knelt down and kissed the sign, then got up and began jumping up and down like a kid. He had just walked 2,160 miles from Georgia to this northern terminus of the Appalachian Trail; it was wonderful to see his joy.

After viewing from the summit for nearly 30 minutes, we started down toward the Cathedral Trail, a shorter but more severe descent route. The Cathedral Trail plunged down a steep boulder-choked gully filled with pink-and-white–Katahdin granite. The rocks were unstable, and even descending the trail was tiring. Hikers struggling up the gully constantly asked us how far away the top was, and how long it would take to get there. We arrived at beautiful Chimney Pond in the shadow of Mount Katahdin at noon.

The final 3.3 miles back to Roaring Brook parking lot took another two hours, and we arrived at our car at 2:10 p.m. The entire hike had taken us eight-and-a-half hours. I noticed as we signed the register on our return that the cutoff time for beginning an ascent of Mount Katahdin from Roaring Brook was 11 a.m. in August. The Class-Day designation, which determines the status of the trails, is also posted here by 7 a.m. Hikers may not proceed above treeline before 7 a.m. if the previous day was determined to be Class IV. (On our hiking day we were all clear to be above treeline before that witching hour.)

I was more tired than I expected to be for a hike of 10 miles, but the reward was an extraordinary view of wilderness from a mountain standing head and shoulders above its surroundings. Kette-Adene may indeed be the greatest mountain in the Northeast.

DIRECTIONS TO TRAILHEAD AND TRAIL ROUTE

To reach the trailhead, take exit 56 from Interstate 95 onto ME 11 and ME 157. Drive northwest about 12 miles to Millinocket, Maine, arriving on Central Street. From the stoplight at Penobscot and Central streets, continue driving west and then north, following the signs to Baxter State Park. The park's visitor center is 16.6 miles from Millinocket. About a mile past the visitor center is the Togue Pond Gatehouse. After the gatehouse bear right on Roaring Brook Road and follow signs 7.7 miles on dirt road to the parking lot at Roaring Brook Campground. This lot has space for 48 cars.

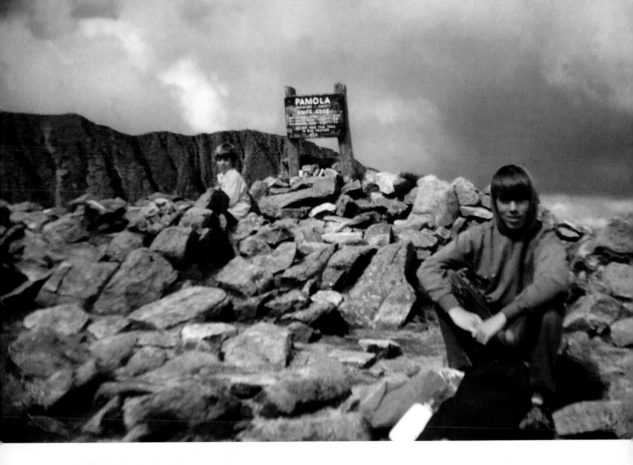

Dan and Tom Bennett at the start of the Knife Edge in 1982

Baxter State Park was a gift from Governor Percival Baxter, who stipulated that the park remain forever wild. The custodians of the park have taken that charge to heart, and today the park remains stubbornly old-fashioned in its regulations and procedures. Entry quotas in Baxter State Park are strictly regulated, and pose a serious problem for the day-hiker. Day use is limited to the parking-lot capacity at each campground. Once the parking lot is filled, no additional vehicles will be permitted. Hikers must therefore arrive at the entrance gate very early or risk being shut out.

Once in the park, permission to climb Mount Katahdin is restricted in other ways. The weather forecast and Class Day for climbing Katahdin is determined each day at 7 a.m., as noted previously. Hikers are encouraged to wait for the Class-Day notification before proceeding above treeline. Any hikers wanting to climb before 7 a.m. can do so at their own risk, but only if the previous day did not receive a Class IV designation. Regardless of conditions, all hikers must register their

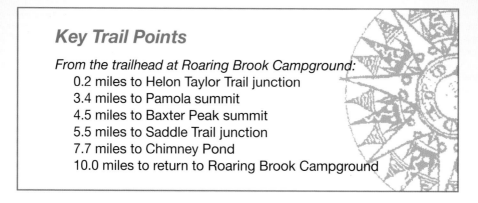

Key Trail Points

From the trailhead at Roaring Brook Campground:
0.2 miles to Helon Taylor Trail junction
3.4 miles to Pamola summit
4.5 miles to Baxter Peak summit
5.5 miles to Saddle Trail junction
7.7 miles to Chimney Pond
10.0 miles to return to Roaring Brook Campground

intentions before climbing. Furthermore, no one may start for Mount Katahdin after noon in June or July, or after 11 a.m. in August, 10 a.m. in September, or 9 a.m. in October. Children under 6 years of age are not allowed above treeline.

After signing the register near the trailhead, head up Chimney Pond Trail. After 0.2 miles, turn left on Helon Taylor Trail. This steep and rugged trail leads 3.2 miles up Keep Ridge to the summit of Pamola at 4,902 feet. The final 1.2 miles of this trail are above treeline, providing the first splendid views of the glacial cirque of the Katahdin Massif as well as the surrounding wilderness.

Follow Knife Edge, a sharp spine of granite barely two feet wide in places, from Pamola over the summits of Chimney Peak and South Peak to the Baxter Peak summit. Knife Edge is precarious in places and will require careful route-finding.

From the summit of Baxter Peak, descend north 1 mile on Saddle Trail to a saddle overlooking Chimney Pond, then descend steeply another 1.2 miles down Saddle Trail to Chimney Pond. Cathedral Trail, which plunges steeply down just 0.2 miles north of the summit, is another possible descent route to Chimney Pond, but it is very steep indeed and is not recommended for descent. Finally, the popular and renowned Chimney Pond Trail returns the hiker along 3.3 miles to the parking lot at Roaring Brook.

WEATHER AND WILDLIFE

Like Mount Washington in New Hampshire, the weather high on Mount Katahdin can be dangerous. Park regulations usually prevent climbing above treeline during bad weather, but hikers must also exercise good judgment. Weather in Baxter State Park can be characterized as highly variable; snowfall can occur any month of the year and temperatures can, and usually do, fluctuate widely. Summer temperatures in the park are usually best in July and August. Fall colors usually begin to emerge in deciduous trees in early September and peak in late September or early October. Lasting snowfall usually begins in mid- to late November.

An incredible variety of animals inhabit the forests and numerous bogs of Baxter State Park. Mammals include moose, deer, bears, otters, mink, martins, fishers, weasels, coyotes, bobcats, beavers, muskrats, raccoons, woodchucks, snowshoe hares, squirrels, and other small rodents. The insatiable blackfly is probably the insect that has acquired the greatest notoriety. The blackfly can make hiking below treeline an extremely unpleasant experience during early summer, so use (and carry extra) insect repellent.

A view from the summit of hikers at the northern end of Knife Edge

LODGING AND CAMPING

Several options for lodging and services are available 16.6 miles away in Millinocket, Maine.

There are ten campgrounds in Baxter State Park. The most convenient ones for this hike are Roaring Brook and Katahdin Stream campgrounds, both open from May 15 until October 15, and Chimney Pond Campground, which is open from June 1 until October 15. Camping reservations must be made only in person or by mail four months prior to the date of the reservation. Requests from Maine residents receive priority on a daily basis. Choice campsites are often taken after only a few hours on any given day. Campground rates are $10 per person, or $20 minimum per campsite.

FEES AND CONTACTS

A fee of $13 per vehicle is charged for each entry into Baxter State Park. This fee is waived for Maine residents. No pets of any kind are permitted within park boundaries, even inside vehicles.

Obtain additional information, including books and maps, from Baxter State Park, 64 Balsam Drive, Millinocket, ME 04462, or by phone at (207) 723-5140. Information is available on the Internet at **www.baxterstateparkauthority.com.**

22 FRANCONIA RIDGE

Location: *White Mountain National Forest, NH*
Distance: *8.8 miles*
Elevation Extremes: *1,770 to 5,260 feet*
Total Elevation Gain: *3,890 feet*
Difficulty: *Strenuous*
USGS Maps: *Franconia 7.5-minute*
Trailhead Coordinates: *N 44° 8' 32.1" W 71° 40' 59.0"*
UTM 19T 0285400 4891173 [WGS 84]

THE BEST HIKE IN NEW ENGLAND

In the spring of 2002, I sent letters and emails to experienced hikers and outdoorsmen in New England, asking them to identify the five best hikes in that region. When I compiled the results, I was amazed! Franconia Ridge had been recommended by all but one person and was identified as the best hike in New England by nearly half of respondents. Never before had I seen such a consensus. It was well-deserved praise. The Appalachian Trail winds 2,160 miles along the spine of the Appalachian Mountains from Georgia to Maine. There are many unforgettable sections of trail along its length, yet most through-hikers identify a narrow ridge in the White Mountains of New Hampshire as the most spectacular part of the route. This is Franconia Ridge, an exposed and stunning 4-mile rib climbing above treeline between Franconia Notch on the west and the Pemigewasset Wilderness on the east.

Fate put me on Franconia Ridge earlier than I expected. On this day I had intended to hike Mount Washington, but mean weather made a shambles of my plans. The Mount Washington Observatory reported a 38°F temperature and 40-mile-per-hour winds at the summit—conditions not to be trifled with. So I drove south to Franconia Notch instead. I knew that Franconia Ridge was 1,000 feet lower than Mount Washington, and I hoped that conditions there would be better. A check with the ranger station at Lafayette Campground confirmed my suspicion. The ridge crest was reported to be very windy, but it was below the cloud deck and was not dangerous. I quickly stuffed food and warm clothes into my daypack, made arrangements to meet my wife back at the trailhead five-and-a-half hours later, walked through the tunnel under the highway, and started up the Old Bridle Path at

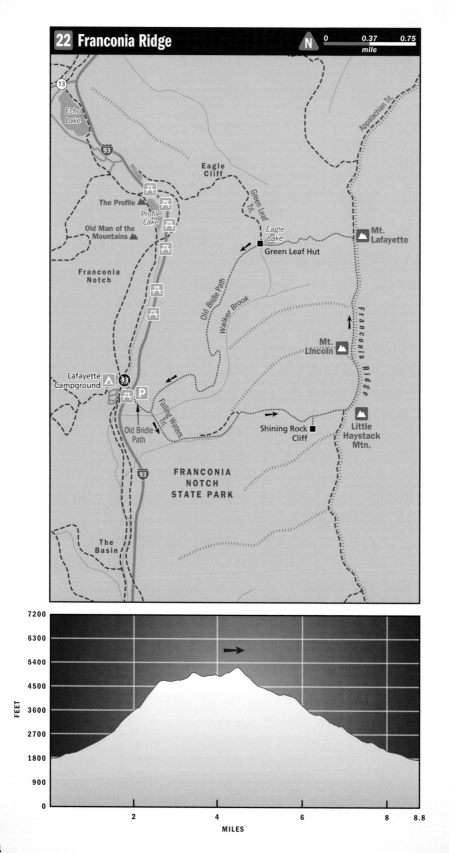

22 Franconia Ridge

N · 0 · 0.37 · 0.75 · mile

13

Echo Lake

93

Eagle Cliff

Appalachian Trl.

The Profile

Profile Lake

Green Leaf Trl.

Old Man of the Mountains

Eagle Lake

Green Leaf Hut

Mt. Lafayette

Franconia Notch

Old Bridle Path

Walker Brook

Mt. Lincoln

Franconia Ridge

Lafayette Campground

Falling Waters Trl.

P

Old Bridle Path

Shining Rock Cliff

Little Haystack Mtn.

93

FRANCONIA NOTCH STATE PARK

The Basin

FEET

7200
6300
5400
4500
3600
2700
1800
900
0

2 · 4 · 6 · 8 · 8.8

MILES

1 p.m. I had never hiked Franconia Ridge before, but I was anxious to see this trail that had been given such stellar reviews.

Most hikers had recommended taking Falling Waters Trail to the top of the ridge, and I soon discovered why. Once I started up Dry Brook, Falling Waters Trail climbed through lovely northern hardwood forest past waterfalls of every size and description. These cascades were especially delightful during ascent, which keeps the waterfalls out in front all the way up. I climbed steadily past Stairs Falls, Sawteeth Ledges, Swiftwater Falls, Cloudland Falls, and numerous other smaller waterfalls. I passed the trail junction to Shining Rock, pressed on to the top of the ridge, and suddenly emerged from the krummholz to arrive at the summit of Little Haystack Mountain at 3:30 p.m.

A powerful gale immediately struck and threatened to knock me off my feet. Franconia Ridge was dark and blustery, but it was below the cloud deck, which rolled swiftly over my head. To the north I could see the shadowy flanks of Mount Washington, but its summit remained buried in the clouds. Mount Washington would have been an uncomfortable and possibly dangerous place. There are many days when Franconia Ridge might have been more comfortable, but it could not have been more dramatic. I put on my parka, hat, and gloves, and turned north on the ridge crest toward Mount Lincoln. There were few people on the ridge, only hardcore hikers, including a few tough backpackers bound for Mount Katahdin in Maine. As I gained elevation toward Mount Lafayette, the wind became even stronger and occasionally I had to hold onto the rocks to keep from being knocked to the ground.

At the summit of Mount Lafayette, I took a final look around at the spectacular view before turning downhill onto Greenleaf Trail at 4:30 p.m. Arriving at Greenleaf Hut at 5 p.m., I took a well-earned break.

After a brief rest, I started back down toward Franconia Notch on the Old Bridle Path. The name Old Bridle Path implied a gentle well-graded stroll back to Lafayette Place, but a horse has not yet been born that could climb this trail with anything on its back! At times the trail followed an exposed and rocky ridge crest that required my utmost attention, especially since the rocks were wet and frequently had water running over them.

Finally the grade eased, and I strolled into the Lafayette Place parking area at 6:30 p.m. I had completed the loop in just 5 hours and 20 minutes. It is a common fault of mine to rush my pace, and this hike clearly deserved more time. The hikers who wrote to me were right: hiking Franconia Ridge is truly a unique and wonderful experience. Together with the Falling Waters Trail, this loop is quite possibly the best day-hike east of the Mississippi River.

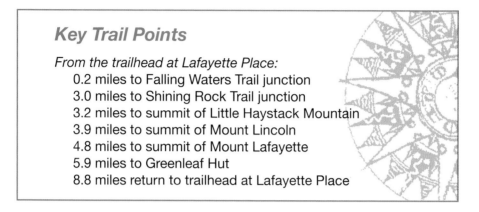

Key Trail Points

From the trailhead at Lafayette Place:
- 0.2 miles to Falling Waters Trail junction
- 3.0 miles to Shining Rock Trail junction
- 3.2 miles to summit of Little Haystack Mountain
- 3.9 miles to summit of Mount Lincoln
- 4.8 miles to summit of Mount Lafayette
- 5.9 miles to Greenleaf Hut
- 8.8 miles return to trailhead at Lafayette Place

The crest of Franconia Ridge

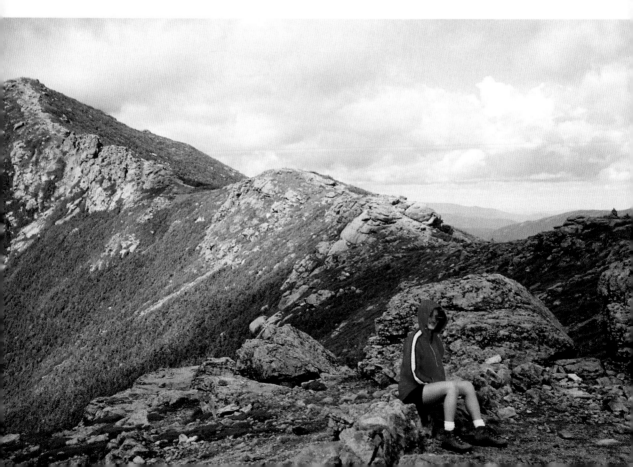

DIRECTIONS TO TRAILHEAD AND TRAIL ROUTE

This loop trail begins from I-93, about 7 miles south of Franconia, New Hampshire. It is the only place I know where an interstate highway narrows down to a single lane in each direction out of respect for its surroundings. Here was the famous profile of the "Old Man of the Mountains" before its collapse in 2003. There is parking for southbound travelers at Lafayette Campground and for northbound travelers at Lafayette Place. A tunnel under the highway connects the two parking lots. Information on the weather and trail conditions can be obtained at a ranger station near Lafayette Campground.

The hike begins on the Old Bridle Path at the Lafayette Place parking lot. After 0.2 miles on the Old Bridle Path, turn right onto Falling Waters Trail and immediately cross Walker Brook. After another 0.7 miles Falling Waters Trail crosses Dry Brook and begins a steep and lovely climb toward the ridge, passing numerous waterfalls along the way. The first waterfall is a beautiful cascade known as Stairs Falls. The trail then crosses to the north bank below Swiftwater Falls before climbing to an old logging road that continues up Dry Brook. At the head of 80-foot Cloudland Falls, there is an overlook with a fine view of Franconia Notch far below. After passing two smaller falls, the trail continues up the stream that flows down from Mount Lincoln. After 1.6 miles Falling Waters Trail swings right, angles uphill away from the brook, and climbs the ridge above via a series of steep switchbacks.

At the last switchback a side trail leads right 100 yards to Shining Rock where there are fine views north and west over Franconia Notch to the Kinsman Range beyond. Finally, Falling Waters Trail enters the krummholz, an area of gnarled and stunted trees just below treeline, and emerges onto the summit of Little Haystack Mountain (elevation 4,780 feet) 3.4 miles from the trailhead.

Turn left onto Franconia Ridge Trail, which is also the Appalachian Trail from here to Mount Lafayette. The next 1.6 miles along Franconia Ridge feature thin alpine soils and fragile vegetation, and hikers are urged to stay on the trail in order to reduce erosion. The portion of the ridge above treeline is exposed to the full force of the notorious White Mountains storms and is very dangerous in bad weather or high winds. Due to the sharpness of the ridge crest, the danger from lightning on Franconia Ridge is especially great. Turn back here if storms appear to be brewing. From Little Haystack Mountain the trail leads north over

Mount Lincoln (5,089 feet in elevation) and to the summit of Mount Lafayette (5,260 feet high) with excellent vistas in all directions.

At the summit of Mount Lafayette, turn left onto Greenleaf Trail and descend steeply to Greenleaf Hut (elevation 3,780 feet). This hut is a good place to take a break. From Greenleaf Hut the Old Bridle Path descends 2.9 miles back to the Lafayette Place parking lot. But don't be deceived, the Old Bridle Path is much more difficult than the name implies. The steep top section is called Agony Ridge, a name coined by those who had to pack heavy loads up to Greenleaf Hut. On the plus side, there are marvelous views down into and across Walker Ravine from several exposed rocky sections, as well as occasional views west to Cannon Mountain, Kinsman Ridge, and Mount Moosilauke. The grade finally relents the last mile or so to Lafayette Place.

Greenleaf Hut on Old Bridle Path

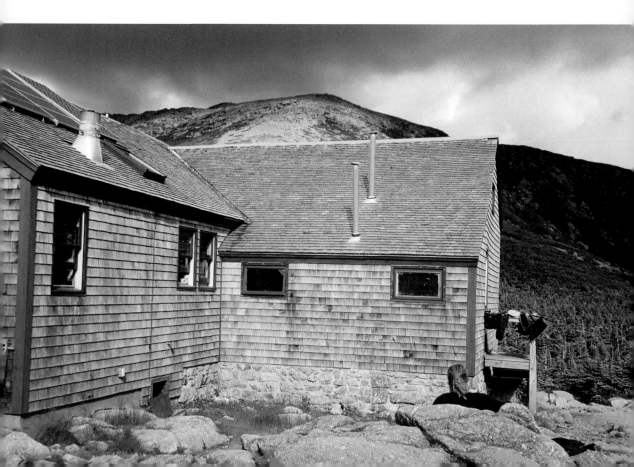

WEATHER AND WILDLIFE

The weather above treeline on Franconia Ridge can be dangerous, although less severe, due to the 1,000-foot lower elevation, than on Mount Washington, 20 miles north. See the description for weather on the Presidential Loop Trail on page 208 for more information.

Wildlife in the White Mountains includes black bears, moose, deer, coyotes, bobcats, beavers, raccoons, woodchucks, and several small rodents.

LODGING AND CAMPING

Lodging and service options are available a few miles north in Franconia and Littleton, New Hampshire.

The Lafayette Campground near the trailhead has 97 campsites with 88 sites by reservation only. Sites are $25 per night and can be reserved by phone at (877) 647-2757 or on the Internet at **www.reserveamerica.com.** The Lafayette Campground can be accessed only from a southbound exit off I-93.

FEES AND CONTACTS

There is a $4 day-use fee for the park ($2 for children ages 6–11).

Additional information is available from Franconia Notch State Park at (603) 823-8800 or at **www.franconianotchstatepark.com.** Information can also be obtained by contacting the White Mountain National Forest at **www.fs.fed.us/r9/white.**

23 PRESIDENTIAL RANGE LOOP

Location: *White Mountain National Forest, NH*
Distance: *9.9 miles*
Elevation Extremes: *3,040 to 6,288 feet*
Total Elevation Gain: *4,510 feet*
Difficulty: *Strenuous*
USGS Maps: *Mount Washington 15-minute*
Trailhead Coordinates: *N 44° 16' 58.4" W 71° 17' 20.3"*
UTM 19T 0317356 4905841 [WGS 84]

A RACE AGAINST THE CLOCK

Early sailors approaching East Coast harbors frequently mistook a shining range of distant mountains for white clouds. These same White Mountains of northern New Hampshire have today become a mecca for sightseers and hikers alike, and no collection of dream hikes would be complete without the Presidential Range. Mount Washington, in the Presidential Range, is the highest mountain in the Northeast and has a well-earned reputation as the most dangerous small mountain in the world. Storms increase in violence with little warning on Mount Washington and its neighboring peaks, and the worst conditions are inconceivably brutal. But for hikers who can wait for good weather, the reward is a dramatic experience in a beautiful alpine setting.

When I surveyed experienced hikers about New England, each included at least one Presidential Range hike, but everyone seemed to have a different favorite. There was no consensus. For my Presidential Range hike I plotted a 9.9-mile loop, including the best of several recommended trails: portions of Wamsutta, Six Husbands, Gulfside, Tuckerman Ravine, Lion Head, and Alpine Garden trails, as well as the summits of Mount Jefferson, Mount Clay, and Mount Washington. Most of the loop is well above treeline and affords dramatic views down into Tuckerman Ravine, Huntington Ravine, and the Great Gulf Wilderness. The trails near the summit of Mount Washington are crowded with tourists, but other portions of the loop remain well off the beaten path.

This was a spectacular and memorable hike, but also a grueling race against the clock. Thanks to the infamous Mount Washington weather, I was running two days behind schedule. On the day I had originally

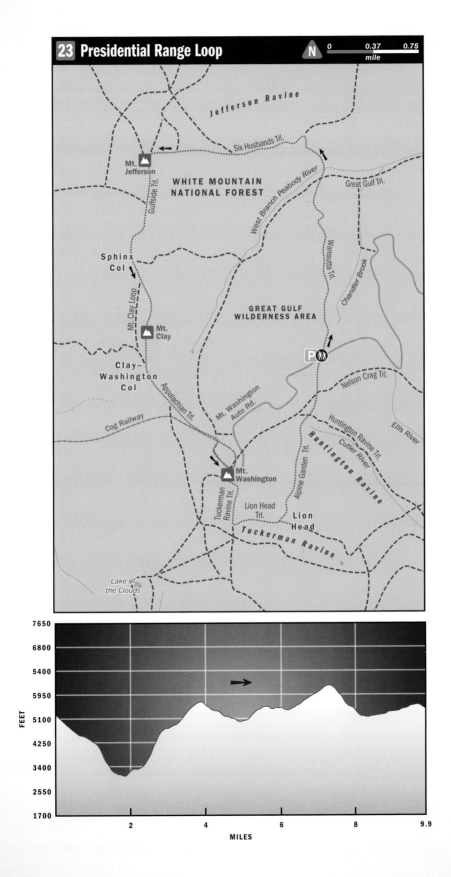

23 Presidential Range Loop

N

0   0.37   0.75
mile

Jefferson Ravine

Six Husbands Trl.

Mt. Jefferson

WHITE MOUNTAIN
NATIONAL FOREST

West Branch Peabody River

Great Gulf Trl.

Gulfside Trl.

Wamsutta Trl.

Chandler Brook

Sphinx Col

Mt. Clay Loop

GREAT GULF
WILDERNESS AREA

Mt. Clay

P

Clay-
Washington
Col

Nelson Crag Trl.

Appalachian Trl.

Mt. Washington Auto Rd.

Huntington Ravine Trl.

Cutler River

Ellis River

Cog Railway

Huntington Ravine

Mt. Washington

Alpine Garden Trl.

Tuckerman Ravine Trl.

Lion Head Trl.

Lion Head

Tuckerman Ravine

Lake of the Clouds

FEET

7650
6800
5400
5950
5100
4250
3400
2550
1700

2   4   6   8   9.9

MILES

planned this hike, the Mount Washington Observatory reported a temperature of 38°F with a 40-mile-per-hour wind and a visibility of only 50 feet—dangerous conditions. By the time the weather improved, I was feeling pressure to do the hike quickly and then rush to Vermont. I thought that I could rip the 9.9-mile loop in six hours, a very rash decision.

It was early August, and the summit of Mount Washington was visible for the first time in four days. I decided to catch the first hiker's shuttle of the morning. The fare charged by the Glen and Mount Washington Stage Company was $22—pretty steep for a one-way ride of only 6 miles. I asked my wife, Mary Fran, to start up the Mount Washington Auto Road at 3 p.m. and to pick me up at the Alpine Garden Trailhead. Unfortunately, the shuttle was 20 minutes late leaving the base, making my already short schedule even shorter.

I left the Auto Road at 9:30 a.m. and started quickly down the Wamsutta Trail. The views into the Great Gulf Wilderness were fantastic. Soon I met three hikers coming up the trail with full packs. "Be

Mount Washington Road and Summit Building

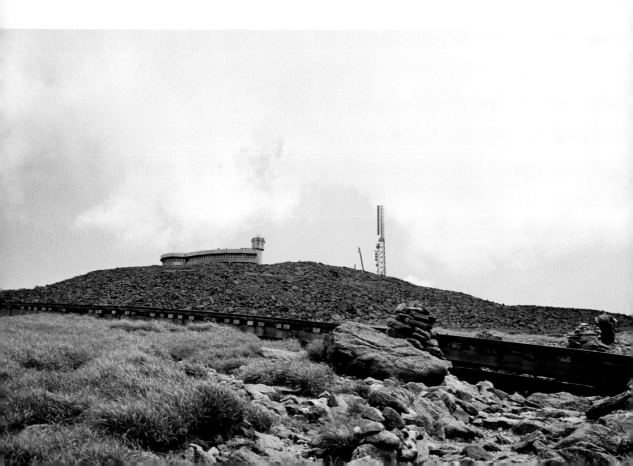

careful below," one said, "it's pretty gnarly!" He was right. The trail plunged steeply down rough boulders into the trees below. It took me a full hour of scrambling to reach the Great Gulf Trail, and I didn't start up the notorious Six Husbands Trail until 10:30 a.m.

The Six Husbands Trail rose gently at first but climbed ever steeper as it approached the north knee of Mount Jefferson. At one point the trail seemed to disappear into a cave under an enormous boulder. I was puzzled until I noticed a small exit tunnel at the back of the cave.

Twice the trail scaled near-vertical rock faces on iron ladders fastened to the cliff. There probably should have been another ladder at the top of the second of these ladders. I found myself rock-climbing up an exposed ridge with the Great Gulf providing considerable exposure. The trail continued above, a delicate connection between rock and sky. I finally reached Gulfside Trail at 12:05 p.m., much later than I had hoped. The weather looked dark and threatening, and I decided to turn left onto Gulfside Trail and bypass the summit of Mount Jefferson.

I moved more quickly along Gulfside Trail and took the loop over the summit of Mount Clay, with stunning views down into the abyss of the Great Gulf on my left. Coming down from Mount Clay, my ears were assailed by a bizarre sound, the high-pitched shriek of a steam whistle. Nothing could have seemed more out of place. Down the mountainside were two steam engines, each pulling three cars, huffing and puffing their way up a minor ridge on the south side of Mount Washington. From this distance they looked like toys. The Mount Washington Cog Railway, an unusual artifact of 19th-century engineering, was completed in 1869 and has been operating more or less continuously ever since. The Mount Washington Cog Railway may be historic and quaint, but it seemed to me a noisy and unsightly intrusion into an otherwise beautiful and natural setting. Gulfside Trail then ran parallel to the railway tracks, and for about 0.5 miles I was treated to the foul smell of coal smoke along with the racket of the beast.

I climbed the summit cone of Mount Washington with dozens of other people streaming down from the summit parking lots like lemmings. Some were obviously ill-prepared for the windy, cold conditions of the day. The summit of Mount Washington, cluttered with people, buildings, antennae, cars, and steam engines, was the least attractive part of the hike. One can scarcely imagine what this remarkable place must have looked like in 1850. I walked into the summit cafeteria at 2 p.m.

I was still running behind my self-imposed schedule, so I bought a sandwich and a soda and, eating as I walked, crossed the parking lot and descended a wooden stairway to Tuckerman Ravine Trail. The trail descended steeply and was filled with tired hikers coming up from Pinkham Notch. I turned left onto Lion Head Trail and arrived at Alpine Garden Trail at 2:40 p.m. I decided not to take the time to divert a few hundred yards down to the Lion Head for the view of Tuckerman Ravine, but instead dashed off toward my rendezvous with Mary Fran on the Auto Road.

Alpine Garden Trail was a joy, traversing a flat grassy area known as a "lawn" adorned with carpets of yellow, purple, and white wildflowers. I felt relieved to be away from the crowds on the summit and alone again with the mountain and the sky. Huntington Ravine was especially spectacular from this vantage point as it plunged steeply down from the Alpine Garden to Pinkham Notch below.

I finally came over the crest of Nelson Crag and looked down at the Auto Road at 3:30 p.m., just when I thought Mary Fran would be there.

The Cog Railroad on the side of Mount Washington

Suddenly, there she was coming up the road. The timing was nothing short of miraculous.

I had achieved my breakneck schedule, but at a great cost. I had sacrificed views from the summit of Mount Jefferson and Lion Head, and had not paused to fully appreciate what the mountain had to offer at any number of beautiful places. Despite my haste, I did experience the drama and splendor of a wonderful alpine setting. A hike through the Northern Presidential Range of New Hampshire is a true American classic.

Key Trail Points

From Wamsutta Trail on Mount Washington Auto Road:
   1.7 miles to Great Gulf Trail junction
   4.1 miles to summit of Mount Jefferson
   5.7 miles to summit of Mount Clay
   7.3 miles to summit of Mount Washington
   8.2 miles to Lion's Head Trail
   9.3 miles to Huntington Ravine Trail
   9.9 miles to the trailhead on Mount Washington Auto Road

DIRECTIONS TO TRAILHEAD AND TRAIL ROUTE

To begin this hike, first drive to the Mount Washington Auto Road at Glen House, about 12 miles south of Gorham on NH 16. The Auto Road, sometimes called the Carriage Road, was constructed in 1855–1861 and is itself a memorable experience. This toll road climbs the Chandler Ridge of Mount Washington in long zigzags, crossing the Appalachian Trail and emerging above treeline after about 5 miles. Just beyond the 6-mile marker on the Auto Road and opposite Alpine Garden Trail is the trailhead for Wamsutta Trail on the right. About 300 feet beyond the trailhead is a small parking area for three or four cars. There will usually be space here since these trailheads are seldom used. Alternatively, a hiker's shuttle can be taken from Glen House to any point on the Auto Road, but other arrangements must be made for the return, because the shuttle will not pick up hikers on the way down. The loop could also be hiked beginning at the summit, but do not hike this loop in the reverse (clockwise) direction, since Six Husbands Trail is not suitable for descent.

From the trailhead on the Auto Road, descend the wild and beautiful Wamsutta Trail, dropping 2,200 feet into the Great Gulf Wilderness.

Just after dipping below treeline, 0.8 miles from the Auto Road, there is an open promontory lookout providing a good view of the magnificent glacial cirque of the Great Gulf. Below this promontory Wamsutta Trail becomes more steep and rugged, finally crossing a small stream and reaching Great Gulf Trail 1.7 miles from the trailhead. Directly across Great Gulf Trail is the beginning of the highlight of the hike—Six Husbands Trail. This wild, rough, and beautiful trail climbs the steep north knee of Mount Jefferson and provides magnificent views of the inner part of the Great Gulf. The trail first crosses a stream, then climbs easily to Jefferson Brook, the stream that flows from Jefferson Ravine. Swinging away from the brook, the trail then winds through a slope containing huge boulders. The trail passes through two boulder caves before attacking the very steep north knee of Mount Jefferson. About 1 mile from the valley floor, Six Husbands Trail ascends a steep ledge on a pair of iron ladders and then climbs under an overhanging ledge on a second pair of ladders. The rock above the last ladder is very steep and could be dangerous if wet or icy. Finally, a rocky promontory is reached at the top of the knee, and the trail begins a moderately difficult scramble up the crest of a rocky ridge. The trail next enters the krummholz, an area of gnarled and stunted trees that manage to survive the violent weather just above treeline. Gulfside Trail is reached after hiking 2.3 miles on Six Husbands Trail and climbing 2,500 feet out of the Great Gulf Wilderness. Gulfside Trail here coincides with the Appalachian Trail.

Cross Gulfside Trail and continue 0.3 miles to the open summit of Mount Jefferson (elevation 5,712 feet), then descend the south ridge of Mount Jefferson to regain the Gulfside Trail. If the weather is threatening, the summit of Mount Jefferson may be bypassed by turning directly south onto Gulfside Trail. This trail is fully exposed to the notorious Mount Washington weather. If weather threatens here, remember that the worst is yet to come and turn back before it is too late.

About 0.3 miles from the summit of Mount Jefferson, the trail crosses Monticello Lawn and descends to Sphinx Col, where there is a view of the Sphinx—a rocky likeness of its namesake—to the left. Above Sphinx Col the trail divides, and hikers may either follow Gulfside Trail or take Mount Clay Loop over the summit (at 5,533 feet) with impressive views into the Great Gulf. The distance is about the same, but the loop over the summit adds about 300 feet of climbing and has the best views.

Mount Clay Loop descends to rejoin Gulfside Trail near Clay-Washington Col (5,390 feet). Just above the col, Gulfside Trail continues southeast between the Cog Railway on the right and the edge of the Great Gulf on the left. If the trail is lost in bad weather, the railway can be followed to the summit. Finally, Gulfside Trail crosses the railway track, joins with Crawford Path, and the two trails turn left and coincide to the summit of Mount Washington.

The summit of Mount Washington provides a welcome respite for hikers—a chance to get in out of the wind, sit down in comfort, and even have a hot meal. Buildings on the summit house a food service, a pack room, a souvenir shop, public restrooms, telephones, a post office, a weather observatory, a radio transmitter, a museum, and facilities for park personnel. Needless to say, the view from the summit with all this clutter is less than pristine.

From the summit buildings, descend south down wooden stairways and across the lower parking lot to Tuckerman Ravine Trail. After 0.4

People on the summit of Mount Washington

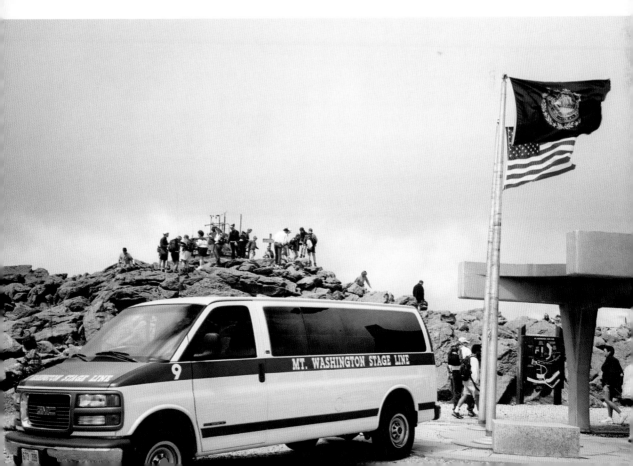

miles from the summit, turn left onto Lion Head Trail. Both of these trails are popular ascent routes from the Pinkham Notch Visitor Center and will usually be crowded. Descend Lion Head Trail, cross Alpine Garden Trail, and continue down Lion Head Trail another 0.2 miles to the Upper Lion Head for spectacular views down into Tuckerman Ravine. Return to Alpine Garden Trail and follow it north toward the Auto Road.

Alpine Garden Trail provides a welcome relief from most of the other rugged and unrelenting trails on Mount Washington. It meanders gently across the wide grassy lawn known as Alpine Garden. The tiny alpine flowers that grow here are best seen in mid- to late June but continue to bloom throughout summer. Especially prominent in this area are white diapensia, the pink-magenta Lapland rosebay, and the very small pink alpine azalea. Hikers are encouraged to stay on the trail to avoid damage to the fragile alpine vegetation.

After 0.9 miles on Alpine Garden Trail, and a little travel off the trail, there is a spectacular view down into Huntington Ravine—a steep glacial cirque equally as spectacular as Tuckerman Ravine. Alpine Garden Trail soon crosses Nelson Crag Trail and then descends gently to the trailhead on the Auto Road.

WEATHER AND WILDLIFE

The worst weather conditions on Mount Washington are ferocious and can materialize with little warning. The summit is under clouds about 55 percent of the time. On an average summer afternoon, the high temperature on the summit is only about 52°F. Winds have gusted over 100 miles per hour in every month of the year and have set a world record of 231 miles per hour. In such conditions it is easy to imagine that safety lies at the summit buildings above, but the safest course is an immediate descent. If the trail is lost high on the mountain, one possibility is to follow the Auto Road or the cog railway tracks to safety. Above all, do not underestimate the danger. The dozens of hikers who have died on these slopes are proof that the weather is sufficiently violent to kill those foolish enough to challenge Mount Washington in dangerous weather.

For wildlife in the White Mountains, see the description under Franconia Ridge Trail on page 199.

LODGING AND CAMPING

The Appalachian Mountain Club (AMC) offers full-service year-round lodging at Pinkham Notch, about 3 miles south of the Mount Washington Auto Road. The AMC also offers lodging in bunkhouses, as well as in eight mountain huts accessible only by trail. Any of these can be reserved by phone at (603) 466-2727. The AMC's Web site is **www.outdoors.org.** Several other options for lodging are available about 12 miles north in Gorham, New Hampshire.

Camping is available at two national forest campgrounds: Barnes Field and Dolly Copp, about 4 miles north of Mount Washington Auto Road at Glen House. Cost is $20 to $30 per site per day (plus taxes and fees). Make reservations by calling (877) 444-6777 or online at **www.recreation.gov.**

FEES AND CONTACTS

The fee for ascending the Mount Washington Auto Road is $23 per car and driver, and $8 for each additional person. Alternatively, The Glen and Mount Washington Stage Company will shuttle hikers up the mountain for $29 (one-way). The phone number for the Mount Washington Auto Road is (603) 466-3988, and their Web site is **www.mountwashingtonautoroad.com.**

For additional information, contact the White Mountain National Forest at **www.fs.fed.us/r9/white.** Up-to-date weather information for the summit can be obtained from the Mount Washington Observatory at **www.mountwashington.org** or by phone at (603) 356-2137, press 1.

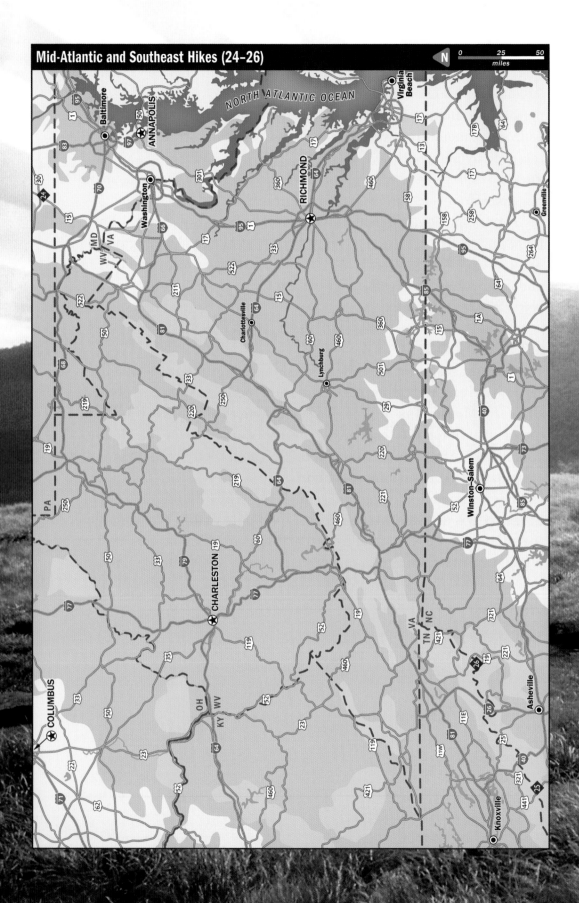

NORTH ATLANTIC OCEAN

Baltimore

ANNAPOLIS

Washington

MD
VA

WV

PA

COLUMBUS

OH
WV

KY

CHARLESTON

RICHMOND

Charlottesville

Lynchburg

Virginia
Beach

Greenville

Winston-Salem

VA
NC
TN

Asheville

Knoxville

N

0   25   50
miles

Mid-Atlantic and the Southeast

24 **BILLY YANK TRAIL**

Location: *Gettysburg National Military Park, Gettysburg, PA*
Distance: *9 miles*
Elevation Extremes: *470 feet to 705 feet*
Total Elevation Gain: *545 feet*
Difficulty: *Moderate*
USGS Maps: *Gettysburg 7.5-minute, Fairfield 7.5-minute*
Trailhead Coordinates: *N 39° 49' 14.4" W 77° 13' 59.7"*
UTM 18S 0308860 4410240 [WGS 84]

AN EMOTIONAL JOURNEY

The April morning dawned gray and somber with a cold drizzle. Heavy fog cloaked the fields and streets of Gettysburg like a shroud, and statues of Civil War soldiers seemed to appear from the mist like ghosts. How unlike that muggy afternoon of July 2, 1863, when troops fought back and forth on these fields, attacking and counterattacking through the choking smoke of battle. The air on that day was filled with the whistle and concussion of cannon shells, buglers and drummers sounding their call, and the screams of wounded and dying men on both sides.

The peaceful fields and farms of Gettysburg today seem far removed from the bloodshed and bravery of that time when a 70,000-man Confederate army under General Robert E. Lee stumbled upon and engaged 93,000 Union troops under General George G. Meade. After three days of carnage, culminating in the attack known as Pickett's Charge, 51,000 Americans lay dead or wounded on the rolling Pennsylvania farmland. Hiking Billy Yank Trail is a trip back in time.

My wife, Mary Fran, and I started our emotional journey along Billy Yank Trail at the Cyclorama Center, first walking south along old Union earthworks to the Pennsylvania Monument, then on to the First Minnesota Monument. Here the men from Minnesota rose up and charged the approaching enemy with little support. The *Gettysburg Heritage Trail Guide,* 12th Edition, offers this account by one soldier who survived:

> Now their cannon were pointed to us, and round shot, grape, and shrapnel tore fearfully through our ranks, and the more deadly Enfield rifles were directed to us alone. Great heavens, how fast our men fell . . . .

The Minnesota regiment successfully held the line here, but at a great cost. Eighty-two percent of the men who went into the battle were

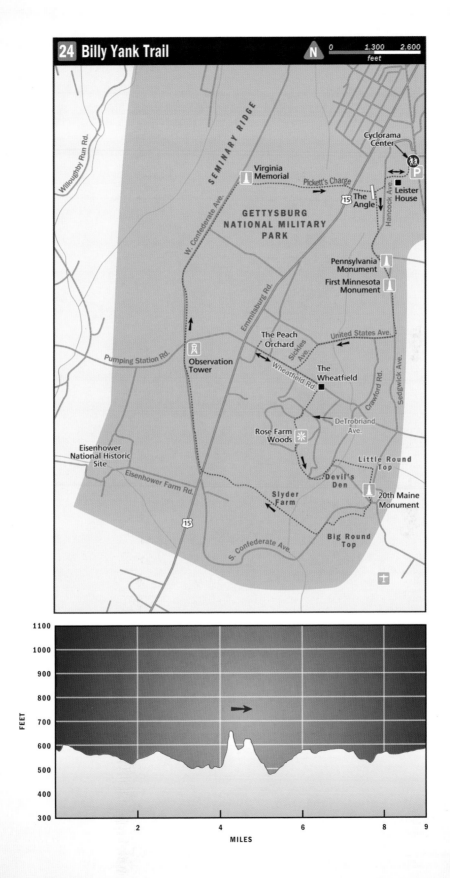

24 Billy Yank Trail

N   0   1,300   2,600
feet

SEMINARY RIDGE

Willoughby Run Rd.

Cyclorama Center

Virginia Memorial

Pickett's Charge

W. Confederate Ave.

15   The Angle

Hancock Ave.

Leister House

GETTYSBURG NATIONAL MILITARY PARK

Pennsylvania Monument

First Minnesota Monument

Emmitsburg Rd.

United States Ave.

The Peach Orchard

Sickles Ave.

Pumping Station Rd.

Observation Tower

Wheatfield Rd.

The Wheatfield

Crawford Rd.

Sedgwick Ave.

DeTrobriand Ave.

Rose Farm Woods

Little Round Top

Eisenhower National Historic Site

Devil's Den

20th Maine Monument

Eisenhower Farm Rd.

Slyder Farm

15

S. Confederate Ave.

Big Round Top

Elevation profile

FEET				
1100				
1000				
900				
800				
700				
600				
500				
400				
300				

2   4   6   8   9

MILES

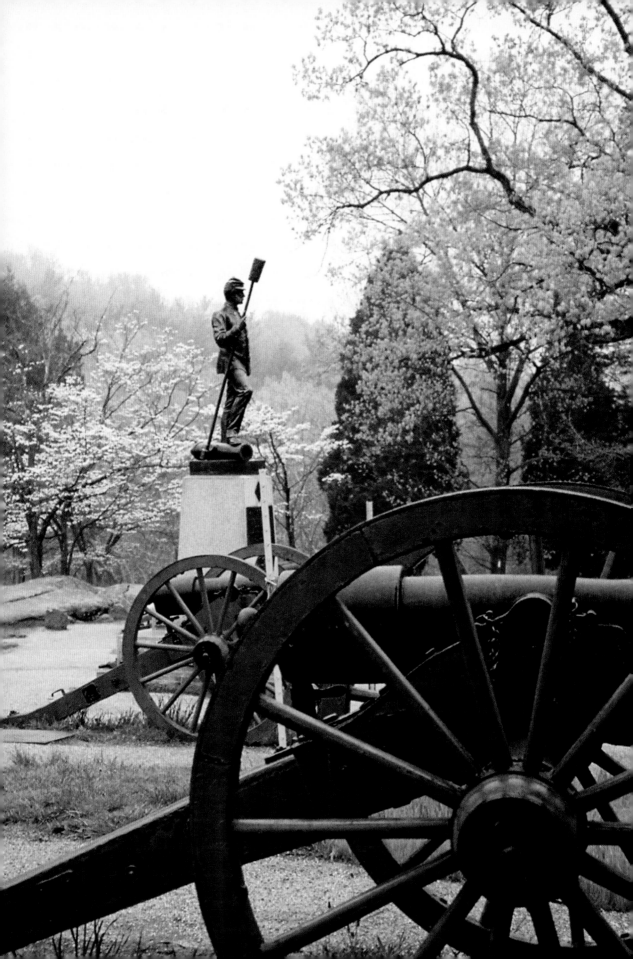

lost. I was overwhelmed by the emotion invoked by this place.

After continuing south on Hancock Avenue then west along United States Avenue, we turned south onto Sickles Avenue to arrive at Peach Orchard after 55 minutes of walking. This orchard was the scene of intense fighting as the Confederate troops under Lieutenant General James Longstreet attacked the southern flank of the Union lines. From here we followed the Union retreat east as they were driven back along Wheatfield Road to The Wheatfield. On July 2, 1863, The Wheatfield was a bloody pool as Union troops fell back under southern pressure. In less than two hours, the field was so covered with the dead and dying that it was difficult to walk across it without stepping on a man. Billy Yank Trail leads straight across The Wheatfield to DeTrobriand Avenue.

After following DeTrobriand Avenue south, we turned left onto a footpath leading through Rose Farm Woods—a lovely and peaceful place. The pink redbuds seemed to glow in the morning fog. But these same woods were the scene of some of the most intense fighting on July 2, 1863, as the southern attack drove Union troops back toward Devil's Den and Little Round Top. We emerged from the woods at the restrooms and drinking fountain near the base of Devil's Den after walking for 1 hour and 45 minutes. If Confederate troops took Devil's Den, it was feared they would have a clear path to Little Round Top above. From here they would hold a commanding position and be able to outflank the Union army. Third Corps troops held Devil's Den as long as possible, but in the end, like their comrades in the Peach Orchard, they were forced to retreat. As they did so, more Union troops arrived on Little Round Top.

Following the path of the Confederate attack, Mary Fran and I remained on Billy Yank Trail up the west flank of Little Round Top to the summit. Confederate artillery on this hill would have had a clear shot at the entire Union line. Here, Colonel Patrick O'Rorke of the 140th New York led a desperate counterattack to hold the left flank of the Union line. Many men were lost, including Colonel O'Rorke.

With each successive attack, the Confederates moved farther right until they encountered the men of the 20th Maine, who were ordered to hold their position at all costs. The 20th Maine repulsed attacks for more than an hour before running out of ammunition. Knowing they could not fail, Colonel Joshua Chamberlain

Now silent cannons of Gettysburg

ordered his men to fix bayonets and charge. The outrageous tactic caught the Confederates off guard, and they surrendered in large numbers. The Confederate attack on the left flank of the Union line had failed.

From Little Round Top, we descended Billy Yank Trail to Warren Avenue and then up the north slope of Big Round Top, around the hill, and down to a parking area on South Confederate Avenue. Just down the avenue, the trail turned onto a footpath alongside a stone wall to Slyder Farm. Past Slyder Farm, the trail continued on to Emmitsburg Road and Seminary Ridge. This was the Confederate battle line on that day. Here, we followed Billy Yank Trail north on West Confederate Avenue along Seminary Ridge, arriving at a prominent observation tower after 2 hours and 50 minutes of walking. The observation tower provides a good view of the battlefield, as well as the Eisenhower National Historic Site on the left.

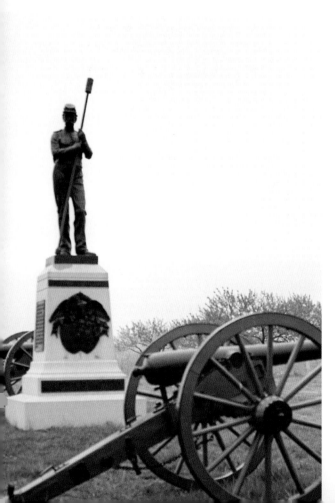

Monuments in the mist at Gettysburg

Continuing along Seminary Ridge, we soon came to the Virginia Memorial and the mounted statue of General Robert E. Lee gazing east toward the Union lines. It was here on July 3, 1863, that Lee, frustrated by two days of heavy fighting and large losses of men, decided to launch a direct frontal assault on the center of the Union line. Lee chose General James Longstreet to lead the attack, but today it is most often called Pickett's Charge after Major General George Pickett, whose troops participated in the advance. The Billy Yank Trail leads straight across the field of that fateful charge.

At about 3 in the afternoon of July 3, 1863, 12,000 southern men emerged from the woods of Seminary Ridge in a line more than a mile long. Less than half that number would return to the ridge where a shocked General Lee watched and waited. Shoulder to shoulder in perfect alignment, they marched toward the Union line, flags unfurled and waving in the breeze. Soon the field was covered with the blinding, choking smoke of battle as cannon fire from Little Round Top pounded the Confederate lines. Still they came. As the attack reached Emmitsburg Road, Yankee infantry rose up and fired into the advancing line of gray. Artillerists in front switched to canisters, blasting thousands of iron balls at close range like shotguns. Only about 400 Virginians reached the stone wall known as the Angle, and those were quickly overwhelmed. Pickett's Charge had failed, and the surviving troops stumbled back to Seminary Ridge. The battle of Gettysburg was over. We reached The Angle, the "high-water mark" of the Confederacy, after walking 3 hours and 50 minutes.

From The Angle we followed Billy Yank Trail and High-Water Mark Trail to the Liester House, which served as General George Meade's headquarters, and finally back to the parking lot at the visitor center. The entire 9-mile hike had taken us four hours, and left a lasting impression on us both. The human drama and tragedy of that fateful day at nearly every stop along this journey was impossible to escape.

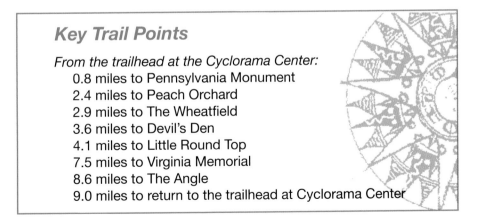

Key Trail Points

From the trailhead at the Cyclorama Center:
0.8 miles to Pennsylvania Monument
2.4 miles to Peach Orchard
2.9 miles to The Wheatfield
3.6 miles to Devil's Den
4.1 miles to Little Round Top
7.5 miles to Virginia Memorial
8.6 miles to The Angle
9.0 miles to return to the trailhead at Cyclorama Center

DIRECTIONS TO TRAILHEAD AND TRAIL ROUTE

No matter which road is taken to Gettysburg, signs will lead visitors to the National Park Service Visitor Center. The visitor center is located between Taneytown Road (PA 134) and Steinwehr Avenue (US 15).

Visitors can purchase the "Gettysburg Heritage Trail Guide," which includes detailed trail directions, as well as commentary, at the park's visitor center for $1. Billy Yank Trail begins at the upper-level (west side) door of the Cyclorama Center, which is 300 yards south of the visitor center.

Billy Yank Trail is part of the Boy Scouts of America Heritage Trails Program. This trail encompasses all of the familiar battle sites of the second and third days of fighting: Peach Orchard, The Wheatfield, Devil's Den, Big and Little Round tops, Cemetery and Seminary ridges, and culminates with a march across Pickett's Charge to The Angle, the high-water mark of the Confederacy. Since the trail route for Billy Yank Trail is intricate, detailed directions are not given here but are described in detail in the "Gettysburg Heritage Trail Guide."

In preparation for this hike, read *The Killer Angels* by Michael Shaara. This captivating work of historical fiction won the Pulitzer Prize in 1975 for its depiction of the Battle of Gettysburg.

WEATHER AND WILDLIFE

Summers in Gettysburg are hot and humid with occasional afternoon thundershowers. Fall and spring are pleasant, with average temperatures in the upper 40s and brisk winds. Winters are wet with occasional snow, which can sometimes force closure of roads and park buildings.

Wildlife seen on this trail is usually limited to gray squirrels, woodchucks, and whitetail deer. Pets restrained on a leash are welcome in Gettysburg National Military Park, but not in park buildings.

LODGING AND CAMPING

There are a large number of options for lodging, as well as private campgrounds in and around the town of Gettysburg. Information regarding lodging is available at the visitor center or by contacting the Convention and Visitors Bureau at **www.gettysburg.travel.** Information can also be found by visiting **www.gettysburg.com.** The only park campground is maintained for scouting and youth groups, and is not available for family camping.

FEES AND CONTACTS

There is no fee for entry or parking in Gettysburg National Military Park.

Address inquires to Superintendent, Gettysburg National Military Park, 1195 Baltimore Pike, Suite 100, Gettysburg, PA 17325. Information can also be obtained at **www.nps.gov/gett,** or by calling (717) 334-1891.

25 ALUM CAVE BLUFF TRAIL

Location: *Great Smoky Mountains National Park, TN*
Distance: *11 miles*
Elevation Extremes: *3,860 feet to 6,380 feet*
Total Elevation Gain: *2,520 feet*
Difficulty: *Strenuous*
USGS Map: *Mount LeConte 7.5-minute*
Trailhead Coordinates: *N 35° 37' 44.7" W 83° 27' 5.4"*
                            UTM 17S 0278004 3945576 [WGS 84]

A NATIONAL PARK CLASSIC

One of the most frightening hiking experiences of my life occurred on Alum Cave Bluff Trail in the spring of 1983. I was climbing with my family to LeConte Lodge (near the summit of Mount LeConte), where we had managed to get reservations for the night. When we reached the heath bald about 2 miles from the trailhead, we surprised a mother black bear with her two cubs. She charged directly at us! We did what we had been told to do—we held our ground. She stopped abruptly about 15 to 20 feet from us, and then ambled off into the bushes. It was only a bluff charge, but it seemed real enough at the time. Now I was again planning to climb Alum Cave Bluff Trail with my family—wife Mary Fran and daughter Jenny—and I didn't want a repeat of that particular memory.

The weather looked ominouson the day of our hike—Easter Sunday. We had booked a comfortable cottage near Gatlinburg, and I nervously watched the weather report as a nasty spring storm bore down on us. I didn't want to tackle Alum Cave Bluff Trail in bad weather, but our reservations for LeConte Lodge that night couldn't be changed. Finally it seemed that the main front would pass, so we went to the trailhead and waited for the rain to stop. Jenny, Mary Fran, and I were on the trail by 12:30 p.m.

The first part of the trail along Alum Cave Creek was as lovely as I remembered. The creek wasn't always visible through the dense evergreens, but occasionally the undergrowth would part to reveal white water cascading over the rocks among lush rhododendrons clinging to the banks. The early mountain people called these rhododendron thickets "hells" because their tangled branches were "hell" to walk through.

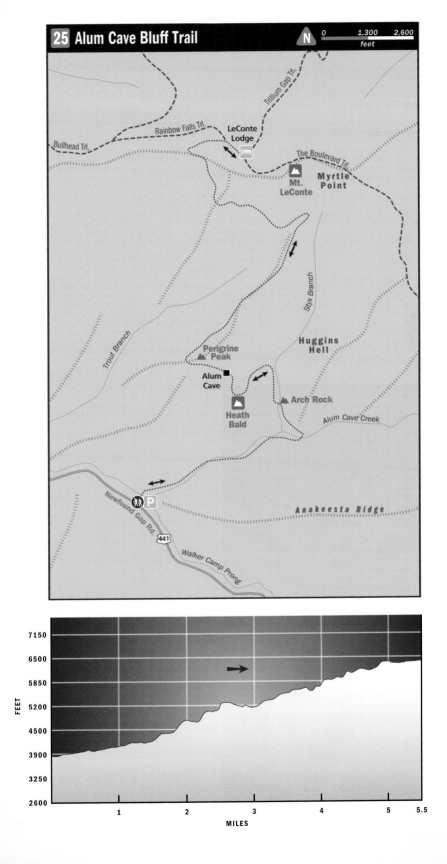

We reached Arch Rock shortly after 1 p.m. and took a break for lunch. It was a beautiful setting with a log bridge spanning the torrent and leading directly to steps climbing into the arch.

After lunch we climbed through Arch Rock and headed up to the open heath bald. The weather was still dark and hazy, but splendid views surrounded us. Below the bald the slope dropped off steeply to the valley of Alum Cave Creek and the West Prong of Little Pigeon River. Mountains soared on every side, including Mount Leconte, Mingus Mountain, Sugarland Mountain, and the twin peaks of the Chimney Tops. To the right was the steep Peregrine Ridge with a tiny hole near the top known as the eye of the needle. Thankfully, there was no sign of bears.

After admiring the stunning view for a few moments, we climbed to Alum Cave, arriving at about 2:30 p.m. After passing through a curtain of dripping water, we found ourselves in an authentic desert where nothing grows. The enormous 200-foot-long ledge extends 50 feet over the trail, completely sheltering the ground beneath, and no springs seep from the dry back of the cave. It's a truly unique environment with a world-class view.

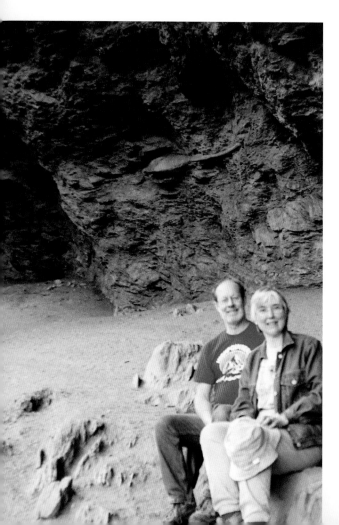

Mary Fran and me at Alum Cave

After a rest in the cave, we pressed on toward the mountaintop. Here the trail became more precarious, and the exposure caused Mary Fran a few anxious moments. The trail climbed narrow ledges, with sheer cliffs dropping below and rising high above. Occasionally the trail crossed landslide scars with uprooted trees and grassy slopes. There was nothing to obscure the views, which extended for miles across the lesser peaks and lowlands of Tennessee.

Finally we passed beneath the huge Cliff Top near the summit of Mount LeConte and crested the top of the trail. A few moments walk through a tunnel of spruce, and we arrived at the cabins of LeConte Lodge at 4:30 p.m. The climb had taken us four hours.

It was good to rest in the cabin we had been assigned and occasionally stroll down to the dining hall for unlimited hot chocolate. But there would be no splendid views and no stunning sunset tonight, as the entire mountain was cloaked in heavy clouds. Dinner was served family-style, with ample portions of soup, homemade cornbread, roast beef, mashed potatoes, and beans. It was a time to share the success of our climb with others at the table, and laughter and good conversation filled the hall. We found the lodge's custom for serving wine to be especially amusing—all you could drink for an extra fee of $5. It seemed that a few guests were trying to get more than their money's worth.

We spent a chilly night in our cabin, because only staff members could adjust the thermostat. But in the morning a hearty breakfast of hot chocolate, coffee, pancakes, scrambled eggs, grits, and homemade biscuits awaited us.

The dark clouds persisted that morning. Everything was heavily frosted, but I was glad there was no new snow, as we would be going back down the steep Alum Cave Bluff Trail. The descent was routine but slow, because parts of the trail were icy. At last, sunshine greeted us as we reached the rhododendron thickets along Alum Creek.

The variety of features, outstanding views, and, of course, the overnight experience at LeConte Lodge make Alum Cave Bluff Trail a true national park classic.

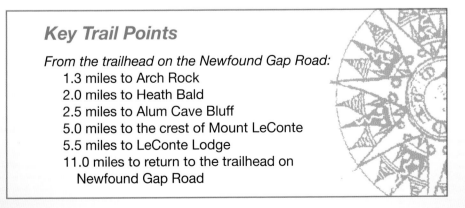

Key Trail Points

From the trailhead on the Newfound Gap Road:
- 1.3 miles to Arch Rock
- 2.0 miles to Heath Bald
- 2.5 miles to Alum Cave Bluff
- 5.0 miles to the crest of Mount LeConte
- 5.5 miles to LeConte Lodge
- 11.0 miles to return to the trailhead on Newfound Gap Road

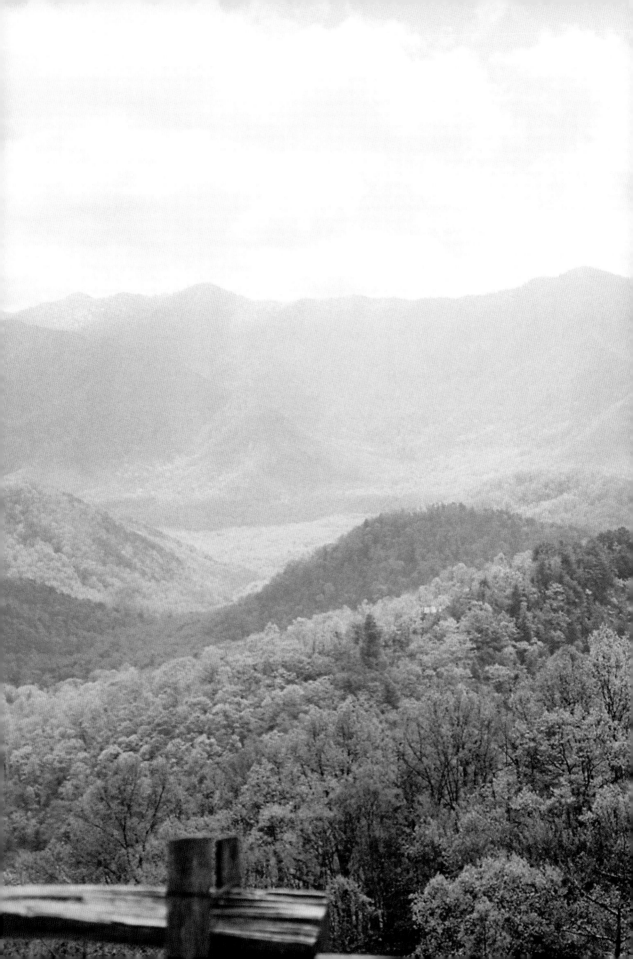

DIRECTIONS TO TRAILHEAD AND TRAIL ROUTE

The trailhead for Alum Cave Bluff Trail is on Newfound Gap Road (US 441) 8.6 miles south of the Sugarlands Visitor Center, or 4.3 miles north of Newfound Gap. The trail begins at a large parking area east of the road.

After crossing a bridge over Walker Camp Prong, the trail winds along Alum Cave Creek through one of the loveliest settings in the Smokies. Giant hemlocks here are more than 200 years old and grow more than three feet thick. The rhododendrons are so thick that at times both Alum Creek and the trail seem to burrow through lush green tunnels. After following Alum Creek for almost a mile, the trail begins to climb along another creek, the Styx Branch, which it crosses three times on crude log bridges. After the fourth log bridge, the trail ascends a curving stairway into tunnel-like Arch Rock. The arch, caused by eons of erosion, resembles the dark turret of an ancient medieval castle.

After crossing another log bridge, the trail passes through a rhododendron thicket, crosses a small stream, and begins climbing a spur of Mount LeConte. The trail climbs steadily until, about 2 miles from the trailhead, it emerges from the trees into an open heath bald. Here the short rhododendrons, mountain laurel, and grasses on a rough outcrop afford one of the best views in the Smoky Mountains.

Past the bald, a tunnel of rhododendron and laurel leads to a rocky shelf with a steel cable for a handrail, and 22 log steps guide hikers up to Alum Cave. The cave is named for tiny traces of alum that are deposited on the interior walls of the cave. Alum was mined here for a time before the Civil War, but the project was soon abandoned because it was not cost-effective.

Beyond Alum Cave the trail ascends a high ledge with steel cables for support. The trail then descends just slightly before climbing the steep slopes of Mount LeConte. This portion of the trail can be particularly hazardous in slippery conditions, and great hummocks of ice bar the way in winter. Finally, the trail curves around to the western slope of Mount LeConte and passes below the huge Cliff Top of the mountain. This is the most precarious and exciting part of the trail.

Finally the trail reaches a crest and turns east through a tunnel of spruce. The trail then joins Bullhead Trail and Rainbow Falls Trail, and the three

(previous page)
Mt. LeConte from Gatlinburg

trails form a continuous path leading to the LeConte Lodge Cabins. Here, hikers can rest before beginning the return trek to the trailhead, or better yet, stay overnight at the historic and classic LeConte Lodge. Hot chocolate and ample meals await those lucky enough to get reservations, and a night in a snug lodge cabin lit by the candle-like flicker of a kerosene lamp is an unforgettable experience. Take the 0.2-mile trail to Cliff Top to watch the sun set over Tennessee, and be sure to take flashlights to light your return in the dark.

After resting or spending a night at LeConte Lodge, return to the trailhead on Newfound Gap Road by retracing the upward journey in reverse.

WEATHER AND WILDLIFE

Great Smoky Mountains National Park receives about 90 inches of precipitation each year, which qualifies the summits as rain forests. This, together with its considerable range of elevation, creates one of the greatest biodiversities in America. Spring is characterized by unpredictable weather, with afternoon showers and thunderstorms common. Sunshine can change to snow in a matter of hours, with the most radical changes occurring in March. Summer is characterized by heat, haze, and humidity, with afternoon showers and thunderstorms common. Daily highs in July and August are typically in the 90s in the valleys. Of course, temperatures are much lower at high elevations, and temperatures above 80°F have never been recorded at LeConte Lodge. Autumn days are typically clear and cool, with the first frost in the valleys occurring in late September.

Whitetail deer are common and obvious in the park. Also fairly common are red and gray squirrels, red and gray foxes, woodchucks, raccoons, opossums, and skunks. Coyotes and bobcats are more reclusive. The black bear, the unofficial symbol of Great Smoky Mountains National Park, is found at all elevations. The bear population in the park is estimated at 1,500, or approximately two bears per square mile. Elk, once eliminated from the Smokies, were reintroduced in 2001 and can be seen in the eastern end of the park near Cove Creek.

LODGING AND CAMPING

LeConte Lodge is the highest accommodation east of the Rocky Mountains and one of the most unusual. The lodge can be reached only by hiking and has no electricity or running water. Like the cabins, the meals cooked on a wood stove are basic but satisfying. Rates are $79 for adults for lodging and $37 for breakfast and dinner. More expensive two- and three-bedroom lodges are also available. Reservations for one year typically begin in the fall of the previous year—with all weekends booked by November. A few reservations are allocated by lottery. For reservations at LeConte Lodge, call (865) 429-5704 or visit **www .lecontelodge.com/reservations.** An overnight at LeConte Lodge requires considerable planning, but it is worth the effort for this national park classic experience. LeConte Lodge is the only lodging inside the park, but a wide variety of lodging and services are available in Gatlinburg, Tennessee, to the north, and in Cherokee, North Carolina, to the south.

Two very large campgrounds are conveniently located for this hike: Elkmont, located west of Sugarlands Visitor Center on the north side of the park, and Smokemont, located along Newfound Gap Road on the south side of the park. Both campgrounds take reservations at (877) 444-6777 or online at **www.recreation. gov.** Campsites in the park run from $20 to $23 night.

FEES AND CONTACTS

There is no fee for entry or parking in Great Smoky Mountains National Park, thanks to an agreement when Tennessee ceded the Newfound Gap Road to the National Park Service in 1930.

Obtain more information from Great Smoky Mountains National Park, 107 Park Headquarters Road, Gatlinburg, TN 37738, or by phone at (865) 436-1200. The park's Web site is **www.nps.gov/grsm.**

26 ROAN MOUNTAIN

> **Location:** *Pisgah National Forest, Carver's Gap to US 19E*
> **Distance:** *13.6 miles*
> **Elevation Extremes:** *3,100 to 6,285 feet*
> **Total Elevation Gain:** *2,490 feet*
> **Difficulty:** *Very Strenuous*
> **USGS Maps:** *Carver's Gap 7.5-minute, White Rocks Mountain*
>   *7.5-minute*
> **Trailhead Coordinates:** *N 36° 6' 22.6" W 82° 6' 36.5"*
>   *UTM 17S 0400070 3996300 [WGS 84]*

A DAZZLING DISPLAY

Possibly the best hike in the southeast, Roan Mountain is especially beautiful during mid- to late June when the famous Catawba rhododendrons turn it into a spectacular jewel of nature. So, I strained to see what view awaited us as we neared Carver's Gap. We had just dropped my son Dan's car off on US 19E east of Roan Mountain, and the vegetation in the valley gave us no clue about the rhododendron bloom on the high balds this time of year. It was mid-June, but I was afraid that we were a bit too early for the peak display. But as we crested the gap, my jaw dropped! A vibrant carpet of pink spread up the balds to the east, and the little parking lot and roadside shoulder was packed full of pilgrims flocking to the spectacle. Each June thousands of tourists travel to Roan Mountain to walk among hundreds of acres of Catawba rhododendrons, which flourish even though truckloads of the rhododendrons were hauled away and sold to nurseries in the 1930s. This is still one of the largest natural rhododendron gardens in the world. Midmorning, we managed to find a parking place and started up the Appalachian Trail through mounds of rhododendron blooms.

Soon, we crested Round Bald and the full spectacle came into view. The slopes of Grassy Ridge Bald ahead were carpeted in pink. Even the trail was covered with blossoms in places. We passed a brilliant orange parade of flame azalea on our right as we topped Jane Bald. I was awestruck!

We crested Grassy Ridge Bald (at 6,285 feet) at 10:20 a.m., and the brilliant flora was complemented by an airy view of the surrounding mountains. Grassy Bald is the only natural 360-degree view above 6,000 feet close to the Appalachian Trail. The Black Mountain chain rose to

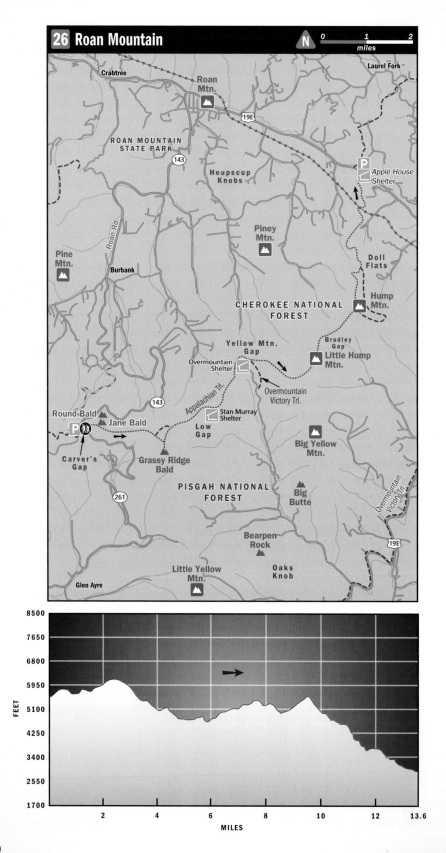

the south, including Mount Mitchell, the highest peak in eastern North America. The distinct shape of Grandfather Mountain dominated the view to the east, and beyond, the distant Piedmont Plateau stretched to the horizon. To the north we could see Little Hump and Hump Mountain, the grassy balds that we would traverse later that day.

There is no feature of the southern Appalachian Mountains more lovely, or more mysterious and inviting than the great "balds" that crown many of its highest peaks. Balds are open mountaintops that occur well below treeline, yet they have remained treeless for as long as history records. How were they originally cleared? Some think that vast herds of elk and bison kept the balds clear by extensive grazing. Others say that Native Americans set fires to keep them open for hunting grounds or religious ceremonies. In any case, the lofty balds of the southern Appalachians serve as a mecca for hikers and tourists alike seeking their airy 360-degree views and unique vegetation.

After enjoying the view for a few minutes, Dan and I returned to the Appalachian Trail and continued north, stopping for lunch at a little campsite just south of the Stan Murray Shelter (formerly known as the Roan Highlands Shelter). Since we were well out of range of the tourists from Carver's Gap, I took our dog Roxy off her leash and let her run. As a mountain cur, an old Kentucky-bred hunting dog, she was clearly in her element.

We paused when we reached Yellow Mountain Gap at 11:30 a.m. Here, hundreds of men from Virginia, North Carolina, and Tennessee under Charles McDowell rode through the snow to meet British soldiers and Loyalists at King's Mountain in 1780. It was a victory that turned the tide against British successes and assured independence for the American colonies. Only a year after the battle at King's Mountain, Lord Charles Cornwallis found himself besieged and forced to surrender at Yorktown. The route of the American patriots was designated a National Historic Trail in 1980 on the 200th anniversary of the decisive battle.

Climbing from Yellow Mountain Gap, we hiked uphill along the edge of a bald that is now becoming overgrown. Soon we came to a view of the climb up Little Hump and, just beyond that, Hump Mountain. We topped Hump Mountain at 3:30 p.m. These balds had no rhododendron gardens, but the views were nearly as good as those from Grassy Ridge Bald. Grandfather Mountain loomed closer, and Mount Rodgers, the highest mountain in Virginia, came into view in the northeast.

After Hump Mountain, it was all downhill as we strolled through the grassy bald now being used for summer pasture. After entering the hardwood forest, we began the long descent toward US 19E. Here, the trail was again carpeted with blossoms, but this time the blossoms were from mountain laurel in the canopy overhead.

The last mile or two seemed long, as we had come more than 13 miles (including a side trip to the summit of Grassy Ridge Bald). We finally came to US 19E at about 6 p.m. We retrieved Dan's car, stopped for a well-earned feast of barbecue pork in the town of Roan Mountain, and drove back up Carver's Gap. This time we headed south from the Gap up toward the summit of Roan Mountain at 6,286 feet. Here the rhododendron gardens were especially dazzling. The fee station was closed since it was evening, so we drove through to the summit and the site of the old luxurious Cloudland Hotel. For 20 years in the late 1800s, guests at the Cloudland delighted in the "pure air and the perfume-laden woodlands" of Roan Mountain. Today little evidence remains of the once grand hotel except the sweet-smelling gardens.

Catawba rhododendron garden on Roan Mountain

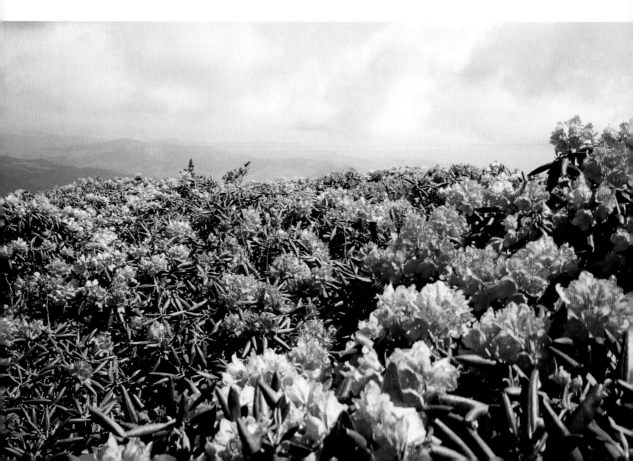

> ## Key Trail Points
>
> *From the trailhead at Carver's Gap:*
>   0.5 miles to summit of Round Bald
>   1.9 miles to summit of Grassy Bald
>   5.1 miles to Yellow Mountain Gap
>   6.8 miles to summit of Little Hump Mountain
>   8.4 miles to summit of Hump Mountain
>   13.6 miles to US 19E

DIRECTIONS TO TRAILHEAD AND TRAIL ROUTE

To reach the trailhead at Carver's Gap from the Blue Ridge Parkway, turn west on NC 226 at Mile 331. Go through Spruce Pine, then turn right on NC 261 toward Bakersfield and Roan Mountain. Carver's Gap is about 26 miles from the parkway. From Roan Mountain, Tennessee, follow CR 143 south past Roan Mountain State Park to Carver's Gap.

The hike begins at Carver's Gap at 5,520 feet and climbs east through Catawba rhododendron gardens on the Appalachian Trail toward the grassy balds beyond. This section of the trail, known as the "Stairway to Heaven," was heavily traveled and badly eroded until it was extensively renovated and stabilized in 2001. After only a few minutes, the summit of Round Bald (5,820 feet) is reached, soon followed by Jane Bald. Views here are stunning but are blocked to the east by the still higher Grassy Ridge Bald. Farther on, the Appalachian Trail veers left to skirt Grassy Ridge, but a 0.3-mile side trail leads right to the highest natural (without structure) 360-degree view over 6,000 feet near the Appalachian Trail. The distant views from Grassy Ridge Bald are spectacular, adding to the already matchless beauty of the extensive rhododendron and azalea gardens.

Return to the Appalachian Trail and descend into the hardwood forest on the northwest flank of Grassy Ridge, reaching the Stan Murray Shelter about 3 miles from Carver's Gap. Continue down through maple, buckeye, and yellow birch to Yellow Mountain Gap and the intersection with Overmountain Victory National Historic Trail. Here the Overmountain Boys—American Patriots from Tennessee, North Carolina, and Virginia—crossed a snowy Roan Mountain on September 27, 1780, on their march to engage and defeat British soldiers and Loyalists at King's Mountain, South Carolina. The Overmountain Shelter is

0.2 miles south from Yellow Mountain Gap in an old red barn.

Continue east and north on the Appalachian Trail along the edge of yet another bald, then climb to summit Little Hump (5,440 feet) and Hump Mountain (5,587 feet). These balds do not have rhododendron and azalea gardens, but still offer spectacular views of the surrounding ridges and the Piedmont beyond. The Appalachian Trail continues north through open, grassy balds, passing through a wooden gate, then again entering hardwood forest. Watch for an easy-to-miss sharp left in a small clearing just beyond Doll Flats. From there the trail descends steeply but is well maintained all the way to Apple House Shelter, about 13.2 miles from Carver's Gap. This shelter is only a few minutes walk along flat path to the trail's end on US 19E.

For hikers who have only one vehicle, a hiker's shuttle to US 19E can be arranged for $25 with the Kincora Hiking Hostel, a popular Appalachian Trail through-hiker hangout in Hampton, Tennessee.

WEATHER AND WILDLIFE

Weather on the high ridges of the southern Appalachian Mountains is highly changeable, especially in spring and fall. Afternoon showers and thunderstorms can occur at any time of year. The Roan Mountain hike is especially exposed to severe weather since it traverses over five balds, and hikers should be prepared. Because of the high elevation of the hike, temperatures in summer are likely to be cool and pleasant.

Whitetail deer are active along the edges of the balds, especially early and late in the day. Red and gray squirrels are common, as are woodchucks, foxes, opossums, skunks, and wild turkeys. Black bears, bobcats, and coyotes are present but more reclusive.

LODGING AND CAMPING

AAA-rated cabins are available at Roan Mountain State Park (**www.tennessee.gov/environment/parks/RoanMtn**) and can be reserved up to one year in advance at (423) 772-0190. Cabins rent from $83 to $99 in season and from $65 to $80 off-season, depending on the day of the week. A few bed-and-breakfast accommodations are available nearby and can be found on the Internet at **www.roanmountain.com**. Several options for hotels and motels can be found a few miles away in Elizabethton and Johnson City, Tennessee.

Camping is available at Roan Mountain State Park, about 5 miles

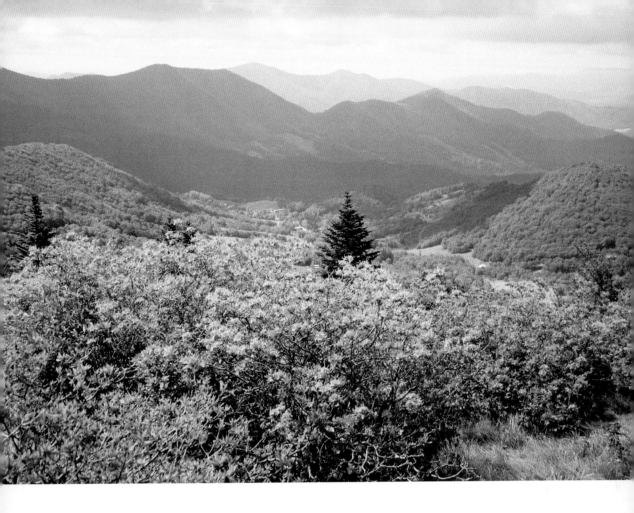

Flame azalea on Jane Bald

north of Carver's Gap on CR 143. The campground has 107 sites that operate on a first-come, first-serve basis for $25 per night.

FEES AND CONTACTS
There are no fees for entry or parking at Carver's Gap. A fee of $5 is charged to drive up Roan Mountain, south of Carver's Gap, from Memorial Day through Labor Day.

Information about trail conditions and the state of the rhododendron bloom is available from Roan Mountain State Park, 1015 Highway 143, Roan Mountain, TN 37687, (423) 772-0190. Information is also available from the Kincora Hiking Hostel at (423) 725-3039 and from the U.S. Forest Service, Appalachian Ranger District, PO Box 128, Burnsville, NC 28714, (828) 682-6146. The Overmountain Victory Trail Association can be contacted in care of the Sycamore State Historic Area, Elizabethton, TN 37643, or online at **www.nps.gov/ovvi.**

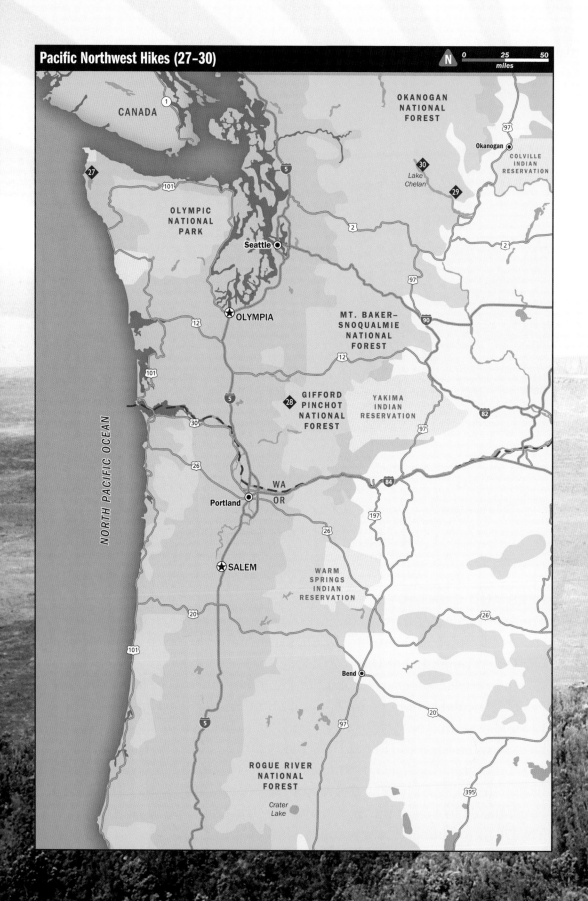

N

0   25   50
miles

CANADA

OKANOGAN
NATIONAL
FOREST

Okanogan

COLVILLE
INDIAN
RESERVATION

OLYMPIC
NATIONAL
PARK

Lake
Chelan

Seattle

OLYMPIA

MT. BAKER–
SNOQUALMIE
NATIONAL
FOREST

GIFFORD
PINCHOT
NATIONAL
FOREST

YAKIMA
INDIAN
RESERVATION

NORTH PACIFIC OCEAN

Portland

WA
OR

SALEM

WARM
SPRINGS
INDIAN
RESERVATION

Bend

ROGUE RIVER
NATIONAL
FOREST

Crater
Lake

Pacific Northwest

27 CAPE ALAVA–SAND POINT LOOP

Location: *Olympic National Park, WA*
Distance: *9.3 miles*
Elevation Extremes: *0 feet to 210 feet*
Total Elevation Gain: *400 feet*
Difficulty: *Moderate*
USGS Maps: *Ozette 7.5-minute*
Trailhead Coordinates: *N 48° 9' 11.1" W 124° 40' 12.1"*
UTM 10U 0375790 5334660 [WGS 84]

SEASTACKS AND PETROGLYPHS

Few places engender more feelings of exhilaration, power, and peace than the rugged coastline of the Pacific Northwest. Waves crash into beaches and headwalls, gnawing away softer rocks and creating seastacks, islands of rock and trees that stand like lonely sentinels offshore. Steep cliffs, crashing surf, driftwood strewn about, and tidal pools teeming with life complete the scene. Unfortunately, such panoramas are becoming less common as civilization encroaches on nature. But the wild shoreline of the Olympic Peninsula remains relatively untouched, and the coast between Cape Alava and Sand Point is rich in both natural and cultural features. Dozens of elaborate petroglyphs, drawn by Makah Native Americans, adorn the boulders between the cliffs and the sea.

Good timing is imperative for the hike between Cape Alava and Sand Point, and timing was not ideal for Mary Fran and me. Two headwalls along the beach can be passed only at low tide, and careless hikers can even be trapped by rising tide. Tide tables for that day in July revealed that low tide would occur at 8 a.m. and 8 p.m., so we would need to hike either in early morning or late evening.

We opted for a late hike, with lights in case we were overtaken by darkness, and departed the trailhead at 3:30 p.m. The ranger at Ozette Ranger Station confirmed that the tide was outgoing and we should have no trouble at the headwalls. The trail to Cape Alava was mostly boardwalk, except for a few stretches of gravel surface, and was pleasant. The trail ambled easily over small hills through forest and low brush. After about 2 miles, a couple traveling the other way warned us of a black

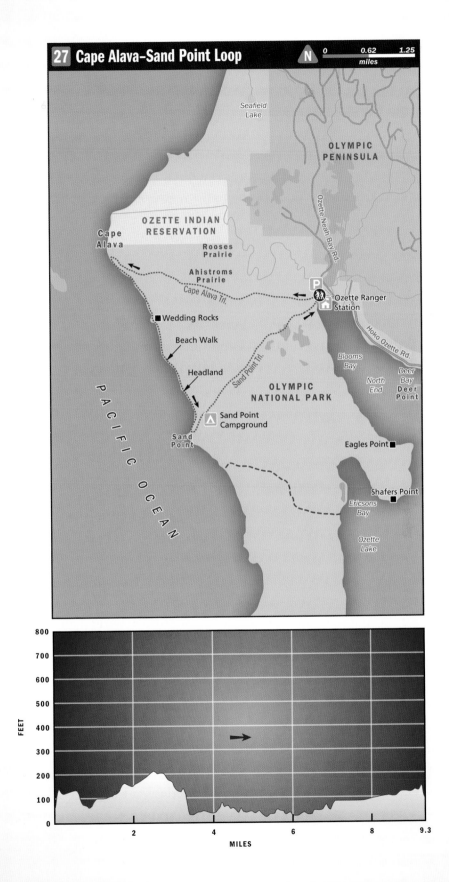

27 Cape Alava–Sand Point Loop

N

0   0.62   1.25
miles

Seafield
Lake

OLYMPIC
PENINSULA

OZETTE INDIAN
RESERVATION

Cape
Alava

Rooses
Prairie

Ahistroms
Prairie

Cape Alava Trl.

Ozette Neah Bay Rd.

P
Ozette Ranger
Station

Wedding Rocks

Beach Walk

Headland

Sand Point Trl.

Hoko Ozette Rd.

Blooms
Bay

North
End

Deer
Bay
Deer
Point

OLYMPIC
NATIONAL PARK

Sand Point
Campground

Sand
Point

Eagles Point

PACIFIC OCEAN

Shafers Point

Ericsons
Bay

Ozette
Lake

800
700
600
500
400
300
200
100
0

FEET

2   4   6   8   9.3

MILES

bear in a clearing ahead. We continued on watchfully but saw no bear.

We reached the coast at 5 p.m. and descended the long grade to the beach. The quiet of the forest was replaced by the sound of waves on the sand and the calls of raucous gulls. Giant seastacks stood offshore, resistant to the relentless attack of the sea. Turning south, we walked on the beach past rocky outcrops, driftwood, and one unlikely surprise: There, among the driftwood, was a large buck lying on the sand. He seemed unconcerned by our presence and watched us passively as we walked by.

After about a mile on the beach, we came to Wedding Rocks—the site of the Makah petroglyphs—which formed a semicircle around the base of a towering cliff. The first petroglyphs looked like frightened faces. As we continued around Wedding Rocks, more drawings came into view—human figures, fish, whales, and fertility symbols. Makah people from Ozette Village, about 1 mile north, probably made the petroglyphs. The drawings have been dated, based on erosion rates, to be about 300 to 500 years old.

We ate a wonderful supper of fruit, crackers, and smoked salmon, which we had purchased on the nearby Makah reservation, in full view of one of the best petroglyphs. It plainly depicted two orcas and two frightened faces. We will remember the peace and beauty of this simple meal in this extraordinary place all of our lives.

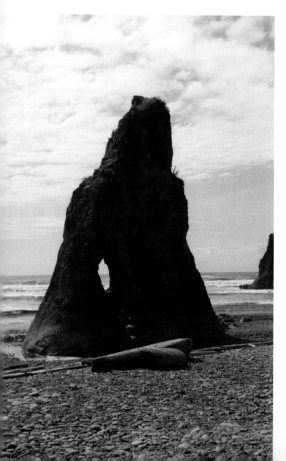

Haystack on the beach near Sand Point

After supper we continued down the beach and around the second headwall. The "trail" over the headwall, to be used in case of high tide, was marked with a circular red-and-black sign. But it did not look like a trail that I would be happy to use. It was nearly vertical, with an old rope dangling alongside it. One look at that trail underscored the importance of hiking this beach at low tide.

Low tide also offered an excellent opportunity to search the tidal pools for an assortment of marine animals, and I explored a few of the pools below the high-tide line. Unfortunately, dusk was quickly approaching, so we hurried on down the beach.

We saw a family camping at Sand Beach and asked about the location of Sand Point Trail, which was not obvious. Once on the trail, we hurried back and arrived at the trailhead near the Ozette Ranger Station in waning light at 8:45 p.m. The Cape Alava–Sand Point Loop came highly recommended from my survey, and it easily met our expectations.

Key Trail Points

From the trailhead at the Ozette ranger station:
3.3 miles to the beach at Cape Alava
5.1 miles to Wedding Rocks
6.3 miles to Sand Point
9.3 miles to return to the trailhead at Ozette Ranger Station

DIRECTIONS TO TRAILHEAD AND TRAIL ROUTE

To reach the trailhead, take US 101 west from Port Angeles, Washington. Just outside Port Angeles, take WA 112 west toward Sekiu. West of Sekiu, take the Mora Road southwest to Ozette. The trailhead starts behind Ozette Ranger Station. Before setting out, check with personnel at the ranger station for trail conditions. While there, pick up information that locates each of the 43 different petroglyphs at the Wedding Rocks site; this material also describes the history and meaning of many of those rock carvings.

As mentioned previously, it is important to time this hike to coincide with low tide. Carefully consult a tide table. Carry a watch and be conscious of the time on the beach—remember that strong winds and storms can significantly elevate the tide levels. The "trails" above the two headwalls are not trails at all, but steep, difficult climbs. If hikers are trapped by an incoming tide, look for the circular red-and-black signs that mark the bypass.

From the trailhead, the trail leads 3.3 miles west to Cape Alava, largely over boardwalk. The boardwalk is slippery when wet, so soft-soled shoes are better than hard-soled hiking boots. Turn south at Cape Alava and walk the beach south to Sand Point, passing the Wedding Rocks petroglyph site and two headwalls along the way. There is no maintained trail on the beach. At Sand Point, locate the return trail behind campsites above the beach and hike back to the trailhead at the Ozette Ranger Station.

WEATHER AND WILDLIFE

The overall weather on the western side of the Olympic Peninsula is a moderate marine climate with pleasant summers and mild, wet winters. On a daily basis, the weather is extremely variable. Rain gear and layered clothing are essential attire. Summers are normally fair and warm, with highs ranging from about 65° to 70°F. July, August, and September are the driest months. Winters are mild with temperatures in the 30s and low 40s, with abundant rainfall.

Wildlife is plentiful on the Olympic Peninsula. Common mammals include beavers, Douglas squirrels, muskrats, coyotes, raccoons, short- and long-tailed weasels, minks, river otters, skunks, black-tailed deer, and Roosevelt elk. Black bears, cougars, and bobcats also make their home in the forest. Olympic National Park protects the largest unmanaged herd of Roosevelt elk in the world. In fact, the park was almost named Elk National Park for that reason.

Common mammals on the coast are river and sea otters, harbor and fur seals, harbor porpoises, and gray whales in spring and fall. Less common marine mammals include sea lions and orca, minke, and humpback whales. Add to these a vast array of tidal pool and tidal zone marine life, including barnacles, mussels, sea urchins, sea anemones, starfish, scallops, limpets, and a variety of crabs.

LODGING AND CAMPING

There are three lodges within Olympic National Park, including Log Cabin Resort, Lake Crescent Resort, and Sol Doc Hot Springs Resort. Each of these offer cabins, motel rooms, and lodge rooms, but these lodges are located several miles from the trailhead. Additional lodging is available in Sekiu; visit **www.sekiu.com** for more information.

Olympic National Park offers 16 campgrounds with a total of 910 sites. The most convenient campground for this hike is the Ozette Campground located near the trailhead. The Ozette Campground has only 15 sites, and the cost is $12 per night. Wilderness camping is also permitted at both Cape Alava and Sand Point. Reservations are required from May 1 through September 30, and may be made in advance

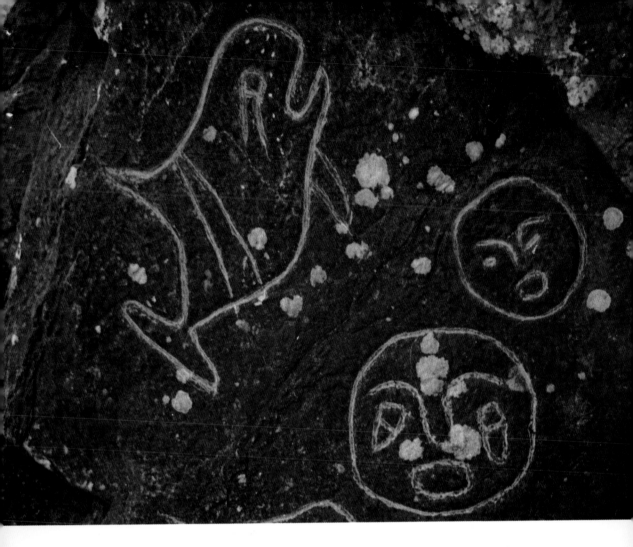

Native American petroglyphs
at Wedding Rocks

by calling the Wilderness Information Center at (360) 565-3100. A permit for the campgrounds on the beach costs $5, plus $2 per person per night. Raccoons and bears are very aggressive and will steal any food left unattended at these sites. Food-storage regulations are strictly enforced.

FEES AND CONTACTS

The fee for entry into Olympic National Park is $15 per vehicle for a seven-day pass.

Additional information can be found on the Internet at **www.nps .gov/olym**. Since heavy rain can cause closure of park roads and facilities, call (360) 565-3131 for a recorded message providing road and closure information.

BOUNDARY–HARRY'S RIDGE TRAILS

Location: *Mount St. Helens National Volcanic Monument, WA*
Distance: *8.2 miles*
Elevation Extremes: *3,890 feet to 4,733 feet*
Total Elevation Gain: *1,900 feet*
Difficulty: *Strenuous*
USGS Maps: *Spirit Lake West 7.5-minute*
Trailhead Coordinates: *N 46° 16' 50.1" W 122° 13' 15.3"*
UTM 10T 0560020 5125510 [WGS 84]

A SLEEPING GIANT WAKES

"Vancouver! Vancouver! This is it!" On May 18, 1980, those were the last words heard from geological survey scientist David Johnson. Then 0.7 cubic miles of debris swept down the north face of Mount St. Helens at speeds up to 730 miles per hour, killing him and 56 others. No trace of David Johnson or his observation post 6 miles north of the volcano was ever found. The lateral blast blew down 230 square miles of forest, and a mushroom-shaped column of ash rose thousands of feet into the sky. Layers of volcanic ash smothered communities in eastern Washington, Idaho, and Montana, where streetlights came on at noon and highway traffic ground to a halt. The ash dusted south into Oregon as well, covering backyard swimming pools in Portland. The eruption of Mount St. Helens was the deadliest and most economically destructive volcanic event in U.S. history.

Climbing the volcano was not allowed until 1986, and in 1990 my son Tom and I hiked up the south side of Mount St. Helens to the crater rim. More recently, I returned to this stunning volcano for another memorable hike.

My wife, Mary Fran, and I began our hike at the Johnson Ridge Visitor Center, near the original site of David Johnson's observation post. We started up Boundary Trail at 11:15 a.m., climbed a hill above the observatory, and then descended to a memorial built to commemorate the 57 people who died here in 1980. We followed Boundary Trail about 1.5 miles east until we came to an overlook. The mountain had experienced a dramatic transformation since I was last there. Grasses, ferns, berries, and a variety of flowers were now thriving in the

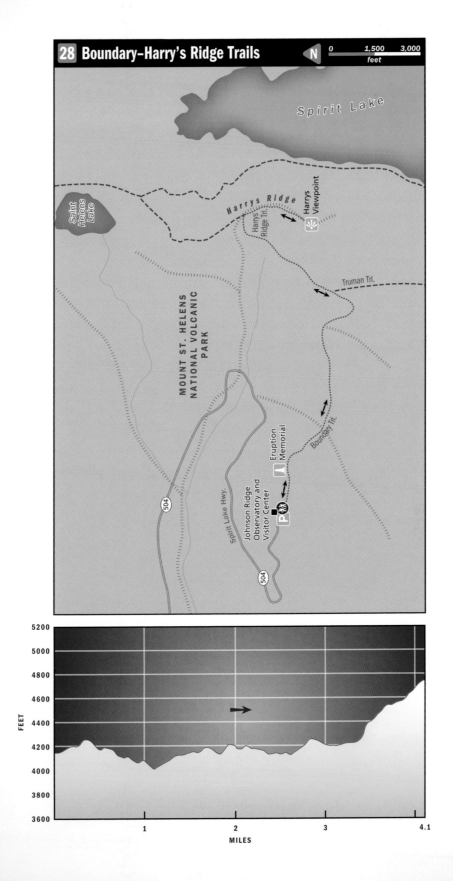

28 Boundary–Harry's Ridge Trails

N

0   1,500   3,000
feet

Spirit Lake

Saint Helens Lake

Harrys Ridge

Harrys Ridge Trl.

Harrys Viewpoint

Truman Trl.

MOUNT ST. HELENS NATIONAL VOLCANIC PARK

Boundary Trl.

Eruption Memorial

Johnson Ridge Observatory and Visitor Center

P

Spirit Lake Hwy.

504

504

5200
5000
4800
4600
4400
4200
4000
3800
3600

FEET

1   2   3   4.1

MILES

once-bleak landscape. Small spruce and willows were already gaining a foothold. A small herd of elk grazed on new-growth buds in the valley below. Following lunch at noon, Mary Fran returned to the visitor center while I kept on toward Harry's Ridge.

After lunch, I continued on Boundary Trail, which descended a steep slope with precarious drops below. As I rounded a point, I finally came in line with the crater and could see, for the first time, the smoldering lava dome inside. The lava dome had grown to the height of the Empire State Building. The weather was not as clear as I would have liked, so the mouth of the crater was only intermittently visible through the passing gray clouds.

I came to the junction with Truman Trail 2 miles from the trailhead. Truman Trail led off in the direction of the crater, but it was closed due to recent volcanic activity. I continued up Boundary Trail to its intersection with Harry's Ridge Trail, turned up Harry's Ridge Trail, and arrived at Harry's Viewpoint at 1:30 p.m.

The view from Harry's Viewpoint was spectacular. The steaming lava dome was more visible, a reminder that the volcano is still unpredictable. Spirit Lake sat directly below.

Before the eruption, Spirit Lake presented an idyllic setting, with crystal-clear waters, lush old-growth forests, and secluded summer

Mount St. Helens in the clouds from Harry's Ridge

cabins and lodges. In Spirit Lake Lodge, the owner, Harry R. Truman, stubbornly refused to leave when the mountain threatened. Like David Johnson at his observation post, Harry and his lodge disappeared without a trace when Mount St. Helens erupted.

Now Spirit Lake still remains a remarkable sight—for a different reason. The north end of the lake had been choked with thousands of floating trees blown into the lake when the mountain was torn apart. When the avalanche from the eruption slammed into the lake, water surged 800 feet up the surrounding ridges, toppling trees and scouring the landscape. As debris from the avalanche came to rest in the lake's bottom, the water level rose nearly 200 feet. Hummocks, giant chunks of Mount St. Helens deposited by the landslide, were still visible in the northern corners of the lake. The devastation of the blast stretched for miles in every direction. I know of no other place where the awesome power of nature is more evident than at Harry's Viewpoint.

My return to the Johnson Ridge Visitor Center was uneventful but no less spectacular. No one knows when Mount St. Helens will awaken again, but the sleeping giant continued to doze for another day, and I arrived back at the trailhead at 3:30 p.m.

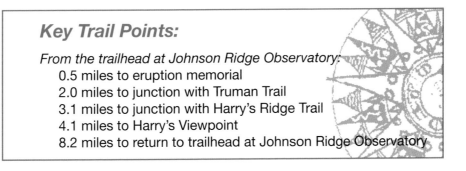

Key Trail Points:

From the trailhead at Johnson Ridge Observatory:
  0.5 miles to eruption memorial
  2.0 miles to junction with Truman Trail
  3.1 miles to junction with Harry's Ridge Trail
  4.1 miles to Harry's Viewpoint
  8.2 miles to return to trailhead at Johnson Ridge Observatory

DIRECTIONS TO TRAILHEAD AND TRAIL ROUTE

To reach the trailhead, turn east from Castle Rock, Washington, at exit 49 on I-5. Follow WA 504 east 47 miles to the Johnson Ridge Visitor Center. It is worthwhile to stop along the way at the Mount St. Helens Visitor Center at Silver Lake for a dramatic presentation of the 1980 eruption. The normal travel time from Silver Lake to the Johnson Ridge Visitor Center is 1 hour and 15 minutes. The trailhead is located at the east end of the Johnson Visitor Center parking lot.

Boundary Trail (#1) leads east along a prominent ridge, then cuts across a slope with excellent views of the blast zone to intersect with Truman Trail (#207). Boundary Trail continues uphill to an intersection with Harry's Ridge Trail (#808). Gain 700 feet up Harry's Ridge Trail to Harry's Viewpoint, and return to the trailhead at the Johnson Visitor Center by retracing the same route in reverse.

WEATHER AND WILDLIFE

The weather at Mount St. Helens is characterized by warm and dry summers, but summer storms are not uncommon. Be prepared for rapid changes in weather and carry warm, layered clothing. Snow is off most of the trails by June, but some late snowpack may remain into July. WA 504 is maintained for winter travel only to Coldwater Lake.

Wildlife has made an excellent comeback since the eruption. Elk and black-tailed deer are commonly seen within the blast zone. Coyotes, red and gray foxes, black bears, gray squirrels, and yellow-bellied marmots are occasionally sighted, with mountain lions and bobcats being less frequent visitors.

LODGING AND CAMPING

There is no lodging or camping within Mount St. Helens National Volcanic Monument. Lodging options are available 47 miles east of Johnson Ridge near I-5 in Castle Rock, Washington. The nearest campground is at Seaquest State Park near Silver Lake and Mount St. Helens Visitor Center. Campsites at Seaquest are $19 to $24 per night and can be reserved in advance at (888) 226-7688 or online at **www.camis.com/wa.**

FEES AND CONTACTS

The fee for entry into Mount St. Helens National Volcanic Monument is $8 per person per day (free for children). There is also a $3 per person entry fee for the Mount St. Helens Visitor Center at Silver Lake.

For additional information, including status of volcanic activity and possible trail closures, contact the Mount St. Helens Visitor Center, 3029 Spirit Lake Highway, Castle Rock, WA 98611. The phone number for the monument headquarters is (360) 449-7800, and the monument Web site is **www.fs.fed.us/gpnf/mshnvm.** If the mountain is quiet, climbing to the crater rim may be allowed. Climbing permits are sold online on a first-come, first-serve basis through the Mount St. Helens Institute.

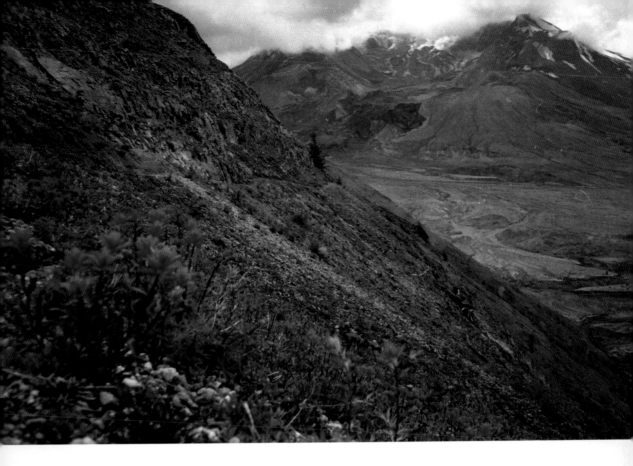

Indian paintbrush on Boundary Trail

29 CHELAN LAKESHORE TRAIL

Location: *Lake Chelan National Recreation Area, WA*
Distance: *7 miles*
Elevation Extremes: *1,096 feet to 1,614 feet*
Total Elevation Gain: *800 feet*
Difficulty: *Moderate*
USGS Maps: *Lucerne 7.5-minute, Sun Mountain 7.5-minute,*
Stehekin 7.5-minute
Trailhead Coordinates: *N 48° 14' 5.2" W 120° 36' 56.2"*
UTM 10U 0677050 5345140 [WGS 84]

THE DEEPEST GORGE

When asked, "What is the deepest gorge in the United States?" most people would reply, "The Grand Canyon." Others with a little more knowledge might reply, "The Snake River Canyon." But both of those answers are incorrect. Glaciers flowing east from the Cascade Mountains of northern Washington have carved an incredible canyon more than 8,000 feet deep. In the bottom of the canyon is Lake Chelan. At 1,500 feet deep, it is the third-deepest lake in America (after Oregon's Crater Lake and Lake Tahoe, on the California–Nevada border). The bottom of the lake has been gouged a remarkable 400 feet below sea level—more than 100 feet lower than Badwater in Death Valley. Granted, the bottom of the canyon is deep under water, but it is nonetheless astonishing.

At the end of the 55-mile-long Lake Chelan lies Stehekin, an isolated community accessible only by floatplane, boat, or foot. Beyond Stehekin, the Stehekin Valley stretches an additional 25 miles deep into the mountains to Cascade Pass. The word *stehekin* means "the way through," since early Native Americans used the valley to travel through the rugged Cascade Mountains for resources and trade. Today Stehekin provides exceptional opportunities for hiking, camping, fishing, and horseback riding in a unique setting. One of the best ways to experience this remarkable gorge is the Chelan Lakeshore Trail. Hikers may walk the entire 17.5-mile trail, or may start at Moore Point for a less strenuous hike.

With my wife, Mary Fran, I boarded the *Lady of the Lake II* at 8:30 on a late July morning. For the next few hours, we rode up Lake Chelan, cruising ever deeper into the mountains as the walls of the gorge

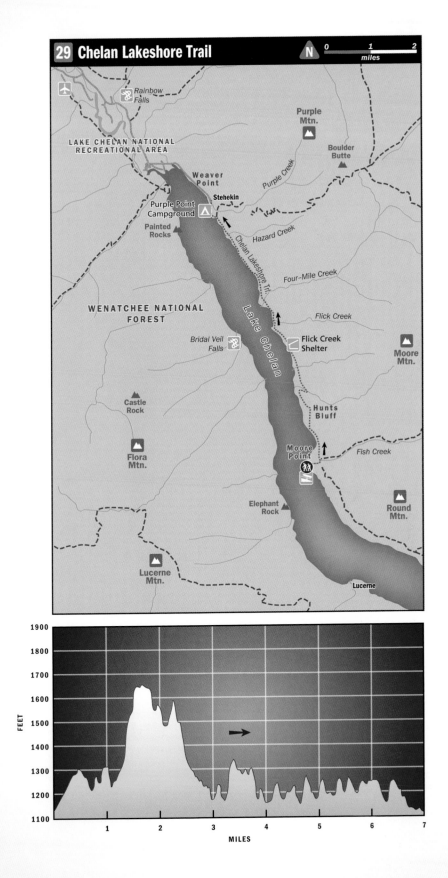

29 Chelan Lakeshore Trail

N

0   1   2
miles

Rainbow
Falls

Purple
Mtn.

Boulder
Butte

LAKE CHELAN NATIONAL
RECREATIONAL AREA

Weaver
Point

Purple Creek

Stehekin

Purple Point
Campground

Hazard Creek

Painted
Rocks

Chelan Lakeshore Trl.

Four-Mile Creek

WENATCHEE NATIONAL
FOREST

Flick Creek

Bridal Veil
Falls

Flick Creek
Shelter

Lake Chelan

Moore
Mtn.

Castle
Rock

Hunts
Bluff

Flora
Mtn.

Moore
Point

Fish Creek

Elephant
Rock

Round
Mtn.

Lucerne
Mtn.

Lucerne

1900

1800

1700

1600

1500

FEET

1400

1300

1200

1100

1   2   3   4   5   6   7

MILES

rose around us. It was a beautiful and relaxing voyage, but I made sure that the crew knew I wanted to disembark at the trailhead for my hike, and the ferry headed for shore at Moore Point. I got off the boat as planned at 12:20 p.m. and waved goodbye to Many Fran. Several other passengers also waved as I walked inland. Once away from the water, the hot air—possibly about 95°F—hit me like a furnace. At the same time I realized that I forgot my water bottle and had only one can of Pepsi to drink over the next 7 miles to Stehekin. I could, of course, drink from the lake at any time, and my guidebook suggested that I could do it, but I don't make it a practice to drink untreated water.

I first looked over the ruins of the fire-destroyed hotel and the historic Moore homestead, with gnarled fruit trees and pastures enclosed by old stone walls. I walked uphill on an old road and passed a sign warning "Beware of Rattlesnakes." I had read that rattlesnakes live here, but hikers are almost never bitten. Nevertheless, the sign made me nervous.

After a short walk uphill, I came to Chelan Lakeshore Trail and turned left toward Stehekin. I was immediately impressed with how dry the landscape was here in the rain shadow of the Cascade Mountains. Dust rose up with every step. The trail soon began a 500-foot climb to the top of Hunts Bluff. The view of Lake Chelan and the canyon was magnificent from the bluff. To the left I could see down the lake to Lucerne and up the lake to Stehekin. Castle Mountain and McGregor Mountain rose to more than 8,000 feet across the lake.

The trail dropped down to the lake at Flick Creek Shelter, and I paused for a late lunch with the sound of waves lapping the shore. I consumed my single can of Pepsi and cursed my carelessness at forgetting my water bottle. After Flick Creek the trail meandered through forest and over creeks, but never again climbed high above the lake, although lovely snow-covered peaks came into view at the head of the valley.

I was feeling very thirsty, so I focused on the end of the lake as my goal. I was pleasantly surprised when I reached Stehekin at 3:40 p.m. about 0.5 miles before the end of the lake. I walked into the first store I came to and drank my fill of Pepsi and juice before I went looking for Mary Fran. She had already checked into Stehekin Landing Resort, where we had a lovely view of Lake Chelan and the deepest gorge in the United States. My hike on the

Lake Chelan from the trail

Lakeshore Trail, with wind-rippled water and sweeping views of lofty mountains towering above, was a masterpiece of American majesty.

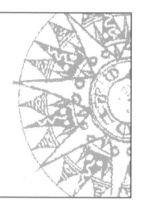

Key Trail Points

From the trailhead at Moore Point:
0.3 miles to Chelan Lakeshore Trail
1.7 miles to Hunts Bluff
3.8 miles to Flick Creek Shelter
4.4 miles to Four-Mile Creek
6.0 miles to Hazard Creek
7.0 miles to Stehekin

DIRECTIONS TO TRAILHEAD AND TRAIL ROUTE

Chelan Lakeshore Trail requires a little planning. Since only one round-trip cruise is offered daily, overnight camping or lodging in Stehekin is necessary. Check the schedule for *Lady of the Lake II* online at **www.ladyofthelake.com** or by phone at (509) 682-4584. Normally, the boat leaves the company dock at 8:30 a.m. and arrives in Stehekin at 12:30 p.m. The boat leaves Stehekin for the return journey at 2 p.m. A round- trip ticket costs $39. There is a faster boat, *Lady Express,* but the cruise up Lake Chelan is a joy and not to be rushed. A round-trip ticket for *Lady Express* is $59. When buying a ticket, be sure to tell the crew where you want to disembark. The complete trail is 17.5 miles from Prince Creek to Stehekin. The hike described here is 7 miles from Moore Point to Stehekin and includes Hunts Bluff, the most scenic section of the trail. If you have reservations at one of the resorts in Stehekin, the resort will pick up your luggage at the dock. Otherwise your luggage will be left at the boat landing and generally will be safe.

From the boat landing at Moore Point, walk a private road uphill 0.3 miles to intersect with Chelan Lakeshore Trail. Follow the trail northwest for 6.7 miles, passing Hunts Bluff, Flick Creek, Four-Mile Creek, Hazard Creek, and Purple Creek along the way.

WEATHER AND WILDLIFE

The weather on the east side of the Cascade Mountains is drier and warmer than on the west side. Summer temperatures in Stehekin reach into the 90s. The average annual precipitation in Stehekin is

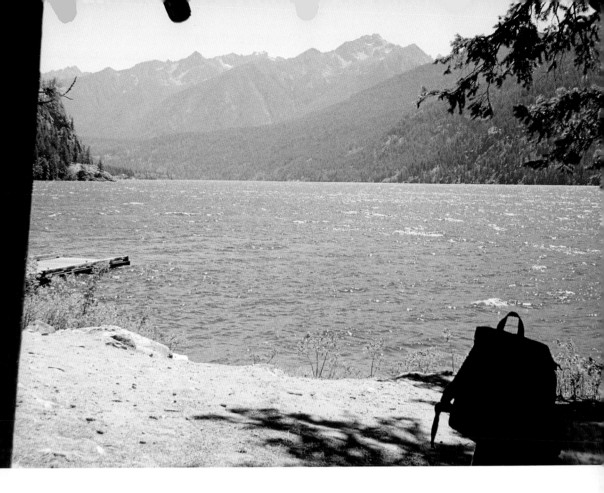

Lake Chelan from Flick Creek Shelter

11 inches. Snow cover from late fall into early spring is expected only above 2,000 feet.

Mammals in the Lake Chelan region include mule deer, wolverines, river otters, cougars, elk, and black bears. Bald eagles are a common sight in Stehekin. We were startled by a bald eagle plunging into the water to fish as we biked along the lake. Rattlesnakes also live along the Lakeshore Trail, but are seldom seen—or heard.

LODGING AND CAMPING

Stehekin Landing Resort (**www.stehekinlanding.com**) lies a short walk from the dock. Reservations can be made via email at info@stehekinlanding.com or by phone at (509) 682-4494. Other options for lodging are in and near Stehekin, and these can be accessed from links on the Internet at **www.nps.gov/lach.** There are numerous options for lodging in Chelan at the eastern end of the lake.

There are two small campgrounds, Purple Point Campground and Harlequin Campground, near Stehekin. Both campgrounds have only seven campsites and are available on a first-come, first-serve basis. Larger campgrounds are available at Lake Chelan State Park and Twenty-Five Mile State Park on the east end of the lake. Campsites at these parks cost $19–$24 for a standard site and $25–$33 for a full-utility site. Reservations can be made online at **www.camis.com/wa** or by phone at (888) 226-7688.

FEES AND CONTACTS

There is no fee for entry into Lake Chelan National Recreation Area. Information for the recreation area is provided on the Internet at **www.nps.gov/lach.** For more information about Stehekin and Chelan Lakeside Trail, contact Golden West Visitor Center, PO Box 7, Stehekin, WA 98852, (360) 854-7245.

30 CASCADE PASS–SAHALE ARM TRAIL

Location: *North Cascades National Park, WA*
Distance: *10.4 miles*
Elevation Extremes: *3,630 feet to 7,610 feet*
Total Elevation Gain: *4,100 feet*
Difficulty: *Very Strenuous*
USGS Map: *Cascade Pass 7.5-minute*
Trailhead Coordinates: *N 48° 28' 29.8" W 121° 4' 30.5"*
UTM 10U 0642262 5370877 [WGS 84]

UNSURPASSED MOUNTAIN MAJESTY

Deep in the heart of north-central Washington lies a land of jagged mountain peaks, massive glaciers, deep forested valleys, and countless cascading waterfalls. This region, designated North Cascades National Park by Congress in 1988, contains some of North America's most beautiful mountain scenery. Few roads penetrate this rugged wilderness, but endless views unfold from trails that lead to flower-sprinkled meadows and high mountain passes. So it was no surprise that when I tallied my surveys, the Cascade Pass–Sahale Arm Trail was rated the best hike in the Pacific Northwest.

On a beautiful Saturday morning in July, my wife, Mary Fran, and I found the trail to Cascade Pass to be well maintained and gradual, gaining about 1,800 feet in 3.7 miles through Douglas fir and Pacific silver fir. As we neared the pass, the trail traversed open talus slopes, and the views began to expand toward Cascade Peak and Johannesburg Mountain across the valley.

We arrived at Cascade Pass at noon and paused for lunch with a view of the jagged peaks on the other side of the pass—Magic Mountain, Trapper Mountain, and Glory Mountain. For the first time, we could see far down the Stehekin River Valley to the southeast. For early Native Americans, this pass was *stehekin,* meaning "the way through" the mountain barrier for trade and resources. Two mountain goats grazed on the meadows near the pass, much to the delight of hikers resting there.

After lunch I continued along Cascade Pass Trail and then turned up Sahale Arm toward Sahale Mountain. Mary Fran decided to linger

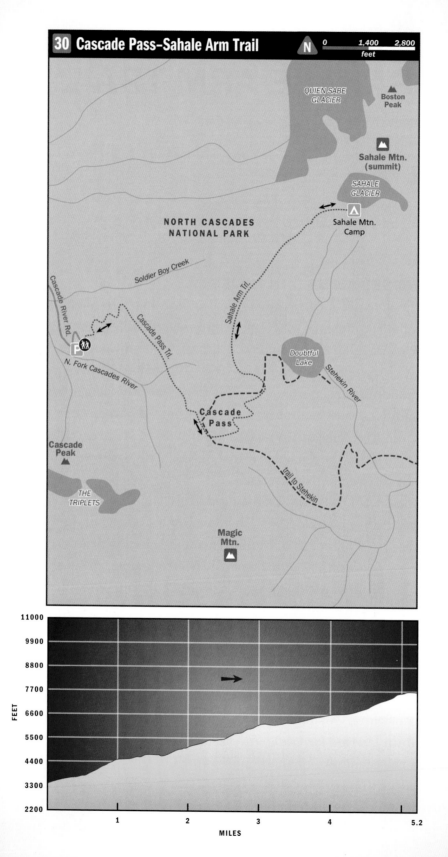

30 Cascade Pass–Sahale Arm Trail

N

0   1,400   2,800
feet

QUIEN SABE GLACIER

Boston Peak

Sahale Mtn. (summit)

SAHALE GLACIER

Sahale Mtn. Camp

NORTH CASCADES NATIONAL PARK

Soldier Boy Creek

Cascade River Rd.

Cascade Pass Trl.

Sahale Arm Trl.

N. Fork Cascades River

Doubtful Lake

Stehekin River

Cascade Pass

Cascade Peak

THE TRIPLETS

Trail to Stehekin

Magic Mtn.

FEET

11000
9900
8800
7700
6600
5500
4400
3300
2200

1   2   3   4   5.2

MILES

at the pass awhile before returning to the trailhead. The trail up Sahale Arm was much steeper and more strenuous than Cascade Pass Trail, and I was concentrating on establishing a rhythm with my pace and breathing. As I climbed high above the pass, I thought I heard a faint cry, "aaakk, aaakk." Perhaps it was the bleating of a distant mountain goat. I climbed higher up the trail. Then I heard it again, "aaakk, aaakk." I stopped to listen more carefully and heard, "Jack. Jack. Damn it. You've got the car keys in your pocket!" That was definitely no goat. After she realized that I had the keys, Mary Fran had been chasing me up the steep slope. I decided at once that walking back down to her would be the prudent thing to do. After trading the car keys for a fuming glance, I was glad to resume my climb up the Sahale Arm above.

As I climbed higher, the views kept getting better. An endless sea of jagged peaks and glaciers rose toward the south. Still higher mountains, Mount Formidable and Spider Mountain, came into view. The trail crested a slope and meandered through mountain heather. Far below, Doubtful Lake, a stunning mountain tarn, added to the beauty.

Farther up the arm, the trail was not maintained and disintegrated into several steep paths. The surface was loose and tiring. The trail required concentration and detracted from the views, which kept expanding as I climbed higher. Finally, I reached a few brightly colored tents nestled in the rocks below the Sahale Glacier. High up on the glacier, some roped climbers were coming down from the summit high above. This was the end of the trail. I sat down for a rest and to enjoy the sight. This was one of the finest mountain views I had ever seen.

I started back down at 2:25 p.m. I could better appreciate the fantastic view on the way down. Far down Stehekin Valley, I thought I could see Lake Chelan where I had hiked only three days before. I kept a leisurely pace and arrived at the trailhead at 5:10 p.m. Fortunately, Mary Fran had calmed down, and I had just hiked arguably the best mountain trail in this country.

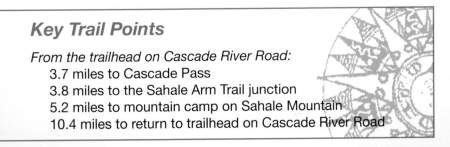

Key Trail Points

From the trailhead on Cascade River Road:
    3.7 miles to Cascade Pass
    3.8 miles to the Sahale Arm Trail junction
    5.2 miles to mountain camp on Sahale Mountain
    10.4 miles to return to trailhead on Cascade River Road

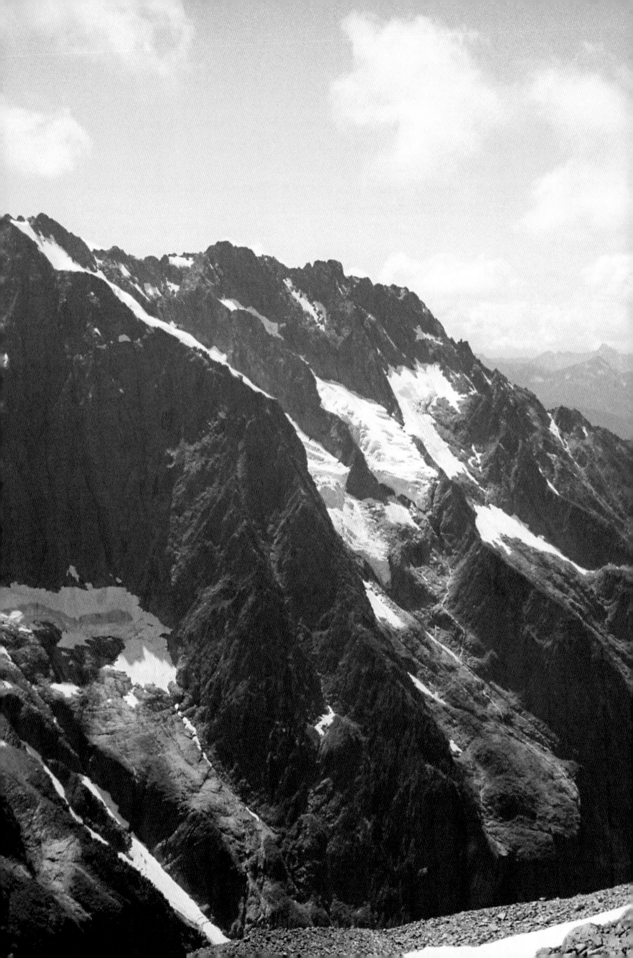

DIRECTIONS TO TRAILHEAD AND TRAIL ROUTE

From Marblemount, Washington, turn south from WA 20 onto the Cascade River Road. Drive southeast on the Cascade River Road for 16 miles to the parking area for the Cascade Pass Trailhead.

From the trailhead, climb steadily on Cascade Pass Trail through a shady forest to Cascade Pass. From Cascade Pass, continue on Cascade Pass Trail, descending slightly on the other side of the pass. Sahale Arm Trail switchbacks up the steep slope on the north side of the pass. The trail relents after it crests the slope and then climbs easily up a ridge above Doubtful Lake. The trail is well defined for a few hundred feet beyond Doubtful Lake. After that, the trail separates into several unmaintained paths that switchback up the rocky ridge above. The trail ends at a small climbers camp at the foot of Sahale Glacier.

WEATHER AND WILDLIFE

As warm, moisture-laden winds collide with the North Cascades, they cool and drop their moisture as rain or snow. The average annual precipitation on the west side of the range is 110 inches. Storms are common anytime of year, and hikers should be prepared with warm, waterproof clothing. The weather is best between mid-July and late September. Heavy snows and rain characterize the North Cascades in winter. As much as 46 feet of snow may fall in winter, and avalanches are common in winter and spring. Snow may persist on the highest trails as late as mid-July.

Conditions in the North Cascades are favorable for a wide array of animals. Three endangered carnivores make their home within the park: the gray wolf, grizzly bear, and Canada lynx. Other species of mammals include black bears, black-tailed deer, wolverines, river otters, cougars, bobcats, elk, moose, and coyotes. Higher up, mountain goats and bighorn sheep graze on alpine meadows, and hoary marmots and pikas are common. Higher still, osprey and bald eagles ride the wind.

LODGING AND CAMPING

Several options for lodging are available in the nearby communities of Marblemount, Rockport, and Concrete.

Looking down on Cascade Pass
from Sahale Arm

Vehicle-access campgrounds convenient for this hike include Goodell Creek Campground and Newhalem Creek Campground near the North Cascades Visitor Center. Campsites are $10 per night at Goodell Creek (first come, first served) and $12 per night at Newhalem Creek (first come, first served) or $21 per night at Newhalem for reservable sites (**www.recreation.gov**).

FEES AND CONTACTS

There are no entrance or parking fees required for North Cascades National Park.

For additional information, write Superintendent, North Cascades National Park, 810 State Route 20, Sedro-Woolley, WA 98284, or phone (360) 854-7200. Information can also be found on the Internet at **www.nps.gov/noca.**

Wildflower meadow above Doubtful Lake

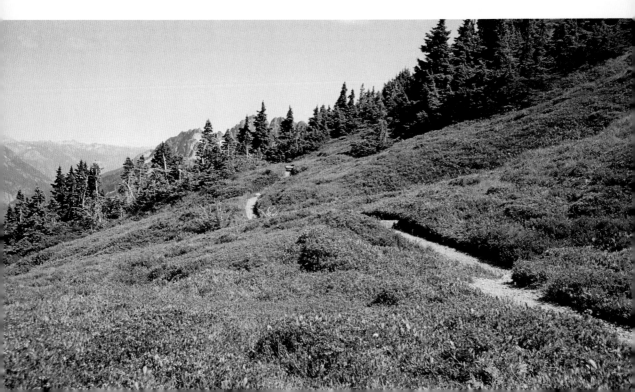

Additional Dream Hikes

Although the following hikes did not make the final cut, they are still some of the most beautiful and significant hikes in America. They include the tallest and oldest trees on the planet, fascinating badlands, world-famous geysers, an intriguing swamp, a unique rain forest, and a plethora of incredible vistas. Those who take the time to walk the *Additional Dream Hikes* below will be rewarded with memories to last a lifetime.

California

PRAIRIE CREEK REDWOODS LOOP
Location: *Prairie Creek Redwoods State Park, Orick, CA*
Trail Route: *Fern Canyon, Friendship Ridge, West Ridge, and Coastal Trails*
Distance: *7.5 miles*
Elevation Extremes: *35 to 640 feet*
Total Elevation Gain: *970 feet*
Difficulty: *Moderate*
USGS Maps: *Fern Canyon 7.5-minute*
Contact: *(707) 465-7347 or www.parks.ca.gov*

Done

METHUSELAH WALK
Location: *Inyo National Forest, White Mountains, CA*
Distance: *4.25 miles*
Elevation Extremes: *9,440 to 10,165 feet*
Total Elevation Gain: *1,000 feet*
Difficulty: *Moderate*
USGS Maps: *Blanco Mountain 7.5-minute*
Contact: *(760) 873-2400 or www.fs.fed.us/r5/inyo*

Southwest

LOST MINE TRAIL
Location: *Big Bend National Park, TX*
Distance: *4.8 miles*
Elevation Extremes: *5,735 to 6,820 feet*
Total Elevation Gain: *1,320 feet*
Difficulty: *Moderate*
USGS Maps: *The Basin 7.5-minute*
Contact: *(432) 477-2251 or www.nps.gov/bibe*

GUADALUPE PEAK
Location: *Guadalupe Mountains National Park, TX*
Distance: *8.4 miles*
Elevation Extremes: *5,835 to 8,749 feet*
Total Elevation Gain: *3,320 feet*
Difficulty: *Strenuous*
USGS Maps: *Guadalupe Peak 7.5-minute*
Contact: *(915) 828-3251 or www.nps.gov/gumo*

BRYCE CANYON LOOP
Location: *Bryce Canyon National Park, UT*
Trail Route: *Navajo Loop and Peekaboo Loop Trails*
Distance: *4.9 miles*
Elevation Extremes: *7,970 to 7,390 feet*
Total Elevation Gain: *1,350 feet*
Difficulty: *Moderate*
USGS Maps: *Bryce Point 7.5-minute*
Contact: *(435) 834-5322 or www.nps.gov/brca*

Hawaii

HALEAKALA CRATER LOOP
Location: *Haleakala National Park, Maui, HI*
Trail Route: *Sliding Sands and Halemau'u Trails*
Distance: *11.3 miles*
Elevation Extremes: *6,850 feet to 9,775 feet*
Total Elevation Gain: *1,460 feet*
Difficulty: *Strenuous*
USGS Maps: *Kilohana 7.5-minute, Nahiku 7.5-minute*
Contact: *(808) 572-4400 or www.nps.gov/hale*

OHE'O GULCH TRAIL (SEVEN SACRED POOLS)
Location: *Kipahulu, Maui, HI*
Distance: *3.7 miles*
Elevation Extremes: *130 feet to 920 feet*
Total Elevation Gain: *790 feet*
Difficulty: *Easy*
USGS Maps: *Kipahulu 7.5-minute*
Contact: *(808) 572-4400 or www.nps.gov/hale*

ALAKAI SWAMP TRAIL
Location: *Koke'e State Park, Kauai, HI*
Distance: *7.4 miles*
Elevation Extremes: *3,685 feet to 4,035 feet*
Total Elevation Gain: *1,100 feet*
Difficulty: *Moderate*
USGS Maps: *Haena 7.5-minute*
Contact: *(808) 241-3444 or www.hawaiistateparks.org/parks/kauai*

Rocky Mountain West

BADLANDS LOOP
Location: *Badlands National Park, SD*
Trail Route: *Saddle Pass, Medicine Root, and Castle Trails*
Distance: *4.2 miles*
Elevation Extremes: *2,414 to 2,648 feet*
Total Elevation Gain: *320 feet*
Difficulty: *Moderate*
USGS Maps: *Cottonwood SW 7.5-minute*
Contact: *(605) 433-5361 or www.nps.gov/badl*

HARNEY PEAK TRAIL
Location: *Custer State Park, Black Hills, SD*
Distance: *6 miles*
Elevation Extremes: *6,145 to 7,242 feet*
Total Elevation Gain: *1,450 feet*
Difficulty: *Moderate*
USGS Maps: *Custer 7.5-minute*
Contact: *(605) 255-4515 or www.sdgfp.info/parks/regions/custer*

GEYSER HILL–MYSTIC FALLS TRAILS
Location: *Yellowstone National Park, WY*
Distance: *7 miles*
Elevation Extremes: *7,261 to 7,445 feet*
Total Elevation Gain: *375 feet*
Difficulty: *Moderate*
USGS Maps: *Old Faithful 7.5-minute*
Contact: *(307) 344-7381 or www.nps.gov/yell*

ICEBERG LAKE
Location: *Glacier National Park, MT*
Distance: *9.6 miles*
Elevation Extremes: *5,010 to 6,240 feet*
Total Elevation Gain: *1,370 feet*
Difficulty: *Strenuous*
USGS Map: *Many Glacier 7.5-minute*
Contact: *(406) 888-7800 or www.nps.gov/glac*

Northeast

BATTLE ROAD

Location: *Minute Man National Historic Park, Concord, MA*
Trail Route: *Old North Bridge to Minute Man Visitor Center*
Distance: *5.5 miles*
Elevation Extremes: *110 to 200 feet*
Total Elevation Gain: *245 feet*
Difficulty: *Easy*
USGS Maps: *Maynard 15-minute*
Contact: *(978) 369-6993 or www.nps.gov/mima*

ALGONQUIN PEAK LOOP

Location: *Adirondack Mountains, NY*
Trail Route: *Van Hovenberg, Avalanche Lake, and Algonquin Peak Trails*
Distance: *11.7 miles*
Elevation Extremes: *2,178 to 5,114 feet*
Total Elevation Gain: *3,200 feet*
Difficulty: *Very Strenuous*
USGS Map: *Keene Valley 15-minute*
Contact: *at www.dec.ny.gov/outdoor/7865.html*

Mid-Atlantic and Southeast

CHARLIE'S BUNION

Location: *Great Smoky Mountains National Park, TN*
Distance: *8.4 miles*
Elevation Extremes: *5,048 feet to 6,030 feet*
Total Elevation Gain: *2,430 feet*
Difficulty: *Moderate*
USGS Maps: *Mount LeConte 7.5-minute, Mount Guyot 7.5-minute*
Contact: *(865) 436-1200 or www.nps.gov/grsm*

OLD RAG LOOP

Location: *Shenandoah National Park, VA*
Trail Route: *Ridge and Saddle Trails and Weakly Hollow Fire Road*
Distance: *7.2 miles*
Elevation Extremes: *990 to 3,268 feet*
Total Elevation Gain: *2,285 feet*
Difficulty: *Strenuous*
USGS Map: *Old Rag Mountain 7.5-minute*
Contact: *(540) 999-3500 or www.nps.gov/shen*

Pacific Northwest

HOH RAIN FOREST
Location: *Olympic National Park, WA*
Distance: *11.4 miles*
Elevation Extremes: *564 feet to 800 feet*
Total Elevation Gain: *250 feet*
Difficulty: *Strenuous*
USGS Maps: *Owl Mountain 7.5-minute, Mount Tom 7.5-minute*
Contact: *(360) 565-3130 or www.nps.gov/olym*

MULTNOMAH FALLS–WAHKEENA FALLS LOOP
Location: *Columbia River Gorge National Scenic Area, OR*
Trail Route: *Trails 441, 420, 419C, 400/420, and 442*
Distance: *6.2 miles*
Elevation Extremes: *130 feet to 1,600 feet*
Total Elevation Gain: *1,480 feet*
Difficulty: *Moderate*
USGS Maps: *Multnomah Falls 7.5-minute, Bridal Veil 7.5-minute*
Contact: *(541) 308-1700 or www.fs.fed.us/r6/columbia*

SPRAY PARK
Location: *Mount Rainier National Park, WA*
Distance: *6.2 miles*
Elevation Extremes: *4,610 feet to 6,140 feet*
Total Elevation Gain: *1,860 feet*
Difficulty: *Moderate*
USGS Map: *Mowich Lake 7.5-minute*
Contact: *(360) 569-2211 or www.nps.gov/mora*

MOUNT SCOTT
Location: *Crater Lake National Park, OR*
Distance: *5 miles*
Elevation Extremes: *3,630 feet to 7,610 feet*
Total Elevation Gain: *1,280 feet*
Difficulty: *Moderate*
USGS Maps: *Crater Lake East 7.5-minute*
Contact: *(541) 594-3000 or www.nps.gov/crla*

Index

DEAR CUSTOMERS AND FRIENDS,

SUPPORTING YOUR INTEREST IN OUTDOOR ADVENTURE, travel, and an active lifestyle is central to our operations, from the authors we choose to the locations we detail to the way we design our books. Menasha Ridge Press was incorporated in 1982 by a group of veteran outdoorsmen and professional outfitters. For many years now, we've specialized in creating books that benefit the outdoors enthusiast.

Almost immediately, Menasha Ridge Press earned a reputation for revolutionizing outdoors- and travel-guidebook publishing. For such activities as canoeing, kayaking, hiking, backpacking, and mountain biking, we established new standards of quality that transformed the whole genre, resulting in outdoor-recreation guides of great sophistication and solid content. Menasha Ridge continues to be outdoor publishing's greatest innovator.

The folks at Menasha Ridge Press are as at home on a white-water river or mountain trail as they are editing a manuscript. The books we build for you are the best they can be, because we're responding to your needs. Plus, we use and depend on them ourselves.

We look forward to seeing you on the river or the trail. If you'd like to contact us directly, join in at www.trekalong.com or visit us at www.menasharidge.com. We thank you for your interest in our books and the natural world around us all.

SAFE TRAVELS,

Bob Sehlinger

BOB SEHLINGER
PUBLISHER